AF757658

MICROBIOLOGY RESEARCH ADVANCES

CONTRIBUTION OF MICROBIOTA TO INNATE AND ACQUIRED GUT IMMUNITY DURING HEALTH AND DISEASE

MICROBIOLOGY RESEARCH ADVANCES

Additional books in this series can be found on Nova's website
under the Series tab.

Additional e-books in this series can be found on Nova's website
under the e-book tab.

MICROBIOLOGY RESEARCH ADVANCES

CONTRIBUTION OF MICROBIOTA TO INNATE AND ACQUIRED GUT IMMUNITY DURING HEALTH AND DISEASE

JOSHUA JOSEPH MALAGO

nova publishers
New York

Copyright © 2015 by Nova Science Publishers, Inc.

All rights reserved. No part of this book may be reproduced, stored in a retrieval system or transmitted in any form or by any means: electronic, electrostatic, magnetic, tape, mechanical photocopying, recording or otherwise without the written permission of the Publisher.

For permission to use material from this book please contact us:
nova.main@www.novapublishers.com

NOTICE TO THE READER

The Publisher has taken reasonable care in the preparation of this book, but makes no expressed or implied warranty of any kind and assumes no responsibility for any errors or omissions. No liability is assumed for incidental or consequential damages in connection with or arising out of information contained in this book. The Publisher shall not be liable for any special, consequential, or exemplary damages resulting, in whole or in part, from the readers' use of, or reliance upon, this material. Any parts of this book based on government reports are so indicated and copyright is claimed for those parts to the extent applicable to compilations of such works.

Independent verification should be sought for any data, advice or recommendations contained in this book. In addition, no responsibility is assumed by the publisher for any injury and/or damage to persons or property arising from any methods, products, instructions, ideas or otherwise contained in this publication.

This publication is designed to provide accurate and authoritative information with regard to the subject matter covered herein. It is sold with the clear understanding that the Publisher is not engaged in rendering legal or any other professional services. If legal or any other expert assistance is required, the services of a competent person should be sought. FROM A DECLARATION OF PARTICIPANTS JOINTLY ADOPTED BY A COMMITTEE OF THE AMERICAN BAR ASSOCIATION AND A COMMITTEE OF PUBLISHERS.

Additional color graphics may be available in the e-book version of this book.

Library of Congress Cataloging-in-Publication Data

ISBN: 978-1-63117-296-0
Library of Congress Control Number: 2014957676

Published by Nova Science Publishers, Inc. † New York

CONTENTS

PREFACE

The large number of microbials in the intestine that overrides the total human cells by ten folds alludes to significant contribution of the microbiota to human health. This is vivid in enteric and some systemic diseases emanating from disruption of the microbiota. The microbiota influences the development and functioning of both, innate and acquired immune systems for gut health. The effect of microbiota spills throughout the various components of the gut immune systems from "primitive" non specific pattern recognition receptors (PRR) to most specific adaptive T cell responses.

To induce immune responses, commensal microbes are recognized by PRRs, which in turn regulate mucosal innate immunity and inflammatory responses. PRRs detect microbe-associated molecular patterns (MAMPs or "infectious non-self") or endogenous "danger signals" derived from stressed, damaged or infected tissue to stimulate the intestinal innate immunity that initiates adaptive immune responses. MAMPs include peptidoglycans, lipoproteins, lipopolysaccharides, teichoic acids, CpG DNA motif, double strand RNA and flagellin. In a balanced microbiota profile, PRR signaling ensures immune homeostasis and protects the host against enteral pathogens. Chapter one of this book will discuss the influence of the microbiota to PRR signaling during health and disease for intestinal immunity.

Chapter two of the book focuses on a second level of innate immune system. This involves cells of the innate immune system that are responsible for driving non-specific innate immunity. They include natural killer cells, mast cells, eosinophils, basophils and the phagocytic cells including macrophages, neutrophils and dendritic cells. However, owing to the great commitment of macrophages and dendritic cells, a separate chapter for these two phagocytic cell types is allocated. Thus chapter two discusses the influence of microbiota on innate cells engendering intestinal immunity under health and disease. It concludes the innate immune system of the intestine.

Macrophages and dendritic cells are professional antigen presenting cells. They sample antigens from the intestinal lumen, process, and present them to cells of the adaptive immune system. Despite of enormous types of enteral antigens ranging from harmful to beneficial, the antigen presenting cells are capable of efficiently discriminating them and driving respective responses to effector cells of the adaptive immune system. While dendritic cells are capable of priming T cell responses, macrophages do polarize the responses. As to how the microbiota influences the functioning of these cells, chapter three is devoted to discuss that phenomenon. The chapter links innate and adaptive intestinal immune systems since macrophages and dendritic cells lie in the interface between innate and adaptive immune systems.

The acquired or adaptive immunity of the gut is split in humoral and cellular components. The humoral immune system is mainly geared by gut-associated lymphoid tissue (GALT) whose components include effector (i.e., epithelial lymphocytes and lamina propria) and inductive (i.e., mesenteric lymph nodes, Peyer's patches, isolated lymphoid follicles, and cryptopatches) sites. It is interesting to note that microbiota influences GALT development and functioning during health and diseases. In germ free animals and those with disrupted microbita, GALT functioning is heavily compromised leading to diseases. Restoration of normal microbiotal profile to such individuals cures the disorders. Chapter four of this book will describe how the microbiota interacts with GALT and other components of the humoral immune system to maintain intestinal immunity under health and disease.

The last chapter, chapter 5, focuses on the second part of the adaptive immune system which is cellular immune system. This system is dominated by several CD4 and CD8 lymphocytes that drive the cellular adaptive immune system. The main components are $CD4^+$ cells which include T helper and regulatory T cells. Other T cells include cytotoxic T, memory, natural killer, and mucosa associated invariant T cells. While T helper cells drive most of the inflammatory responses, regulatory T cells downregulate these responses. As such, they are considered potential therapeutic agents of the future. Current knowledge indicates that the functioning of most, if not all, T cells is influenced by the microbiota. Chapter 5 is therefore devoted to discuss how the microbiota interacts with T cells during health and disease to foster intestinal immunity.

In the past few years we have encountered mounting evidence showing that the microbiota plays essential role in regulating and maintaining host's intestinal immunity. This is done through various ways including; regulation of mucin gene expression by goblet cells, modification of glycosylation of mucus to interfere with bacterial adhesion, colonization and invasion, induction of secretion of antimicrobial peptides by intestinal Paneth cells, regulation of alterations of intestinal permeability caused by infection, stress, and inflammation, and influences on development of mucosal and systemic immunity. It is becoming well comprehended that microbiota is pivotal to the intestinal immunity through crosstalk with the epithelium, immune cells and the immune system in general. Disruption of microbiota balance often leads to disease. This book explores recent findings on how microbiota influences the intestinal immune responses, both innate and adaptive, to foster the intestinal mucosal immunity. The insight gained could contribute to designing approaches suitable for treating gastrointestinal diseases caused by disruption of the microbiota.

Chapter 1

INFLUENCE OF MICROBIOTA TO PATTERN RECOGNITION RECEPTOR SIGNALING FOR INTESTINAL IMMUNITY

ABSTRACT

The contribution of intestinal epithelium to the innate immune system includes detecting luminal microbes, transducing signals, and activating inflammatory mediator release by epithelial and other cells of the immune system like the antigen presenting cells. Microbial antigens are detected by cells of the innate immune system through their pattern recognition receptors (PRRs). The PRRs recognize microbe-associated molecular patterns and generate signals that activate transcription pathways like nuclear factor kappa B and mitogen activated protein kinases. This activation leads to production of inflammatory and growth mediators that drive the immune system to elicit tolerance or immune response designated at maintaining immune homeostasis. Key to this signaling is the gut microbiota. Intestinal epithelial cell sensing of optimally balanced microbiota favors immune homeostasis whereas sensing under disrupted microbiota impairs immune function and predisposes to disease. Understanding the PRR-microbiota signaling would be useful in designing therapeutics for various immune-mediated disorders caused by imbalances of microbiota.

INTRODUCTION

Microorganisms and other noxious agents that successfully enter the gastrointestinal tract encounter intestinal physicochemical barrier as well as cells and mechanisms of innate immune system. In order for them to establish in the gut and cause disease, they must cross these elements. The exposure of intestinal epithelial cells (IECs) to this wide range of enteral agents triggers highly controlled responses to effect appropriate functions. Usually the responses involve elimination of the microorganisms or neutralization of toxins and other agents. To meet this function, IECs recognize antigens and respond by synthesizing a wide range of products including pro- and anti-inflammatory mediators, mucus, and antimicrobials (Lee et al., 2006; Malago 2014). They also transmit signals to underlying cells in the mucosa to drive the desired responses (DePaolo et al., 2012; Pickard et al., 2014).

Despite of enormous diversity in enteral antigens, the innate immune system is capable of discriminating potential pathogens from beneficial microbiota through a restricted number of preformed receptors named the pattern recognition receptors (PRR). They include membrane-bound toll-like receptors (TLR) and cytoplasmic nucleotide oligomerization domain (NOD)-like receptors (NLR). A series of TLR (including TLR1, 2, 3, 4, 5, 9) and NOD1/2 receptors are expressed by IECs to recognize motifs conserved by bacteria but not higher eukaryotes (Medzhitov 2007; Barton and Kagan 2009; Franchi et al., 2009; Langefeld et al., 2009; Wagner 2012; Kamdar et al., 2013; Kant et al., 2013). The expression may also follow recognition of damaged, injured or stressed cells that send out alarm signals that are recognized by the same receptors as those for pathogens (Matzinger 2002). Innate response is usually triggered when microbes are identified by the PRR which allows immediate recognition of bacteria and rapid response by cells of the innate immune system (Langefeld et al., 2009; Wagner 2012; Kamdar et al., 2013; Kant et al., 2013). Endocytic PRRs are involved in phagocytosis without relaying intracellular signals. They recognize receptors on phagocytes such as macrophages to clear apoptotic cells (Jeannin et al., 2008).

Signaling through PRR system generates transmembrane signals on cell surface that transduce the signals through kinase enzymes before activating putative transcription pathways like nuclear factor kappa B (NF-κB) and mitogen activated protein kinase (MAPK) (Figure 1) (Malago et al., 2002; Zhong et al., 2007) Activation of NF-κB drives transcription of a series of genes coding for inflammatory cytokines, enzymes and growth factors

(Malago et al., 2002). Important end results of NF-κB products to innate immune system are pro-inflammatory cytokines, especially chemoattractants like interleukin (IL)-8 and tumor necrosis factor (TNF)-α that attract inflammatory cells, particularly neutrophils, to the site of insult. The NF-κB activation also leads to generation of nitric oxide that imparts its antimicrobial activity. Part of this signaling activates cells underlying lamina propria (LP) including a population of innate lymphoid cells (ILCs) (Figure 2). The activated ILCs produce effector cytokines essential for protective and pathogenic roles during intestinal inflammation (Schenten and Medzhitov 2011). It is the LP dendritic cells (DCs) that determine whether anti- or pro-inflammatory response should be elicited in response to a particular antigen.

The influence of microbiota to the PRR signaling is evident. It activates and shapes the downstream responses of PRR signaling to maintain gut immunity (Bermudez-Brito et al., 2014; Yu et al., 2014). To meet this function, the microbiota drives PRR signaling to generate immune homeostasis in a steady state gut environment and induce immune responses to combat and eliminate noxious agents and restore immunity during perturbations. Disruption of the microbiota fails the signaling optimal performance and often leads to immune mediated disorders like inflammatory bowel disease and colorectal cancers (Song et al., 2014; Yu et al., 2014). Similarly, chemical colitis animal models show a decrease in protective bacteria but an increase in aggressive bacteria. They also show a decrease in the richness and diversity of both mucosal and luminal microbiota. These changes correlate with the severity of colitis as well as the expression of PRR (Xue et al., 2013). The expression of PRR in such animals is pivotal to the development of colitis. Indeed, the microbiota effect on PRR signaling is pertinent for gut immunity. It is therefore compelling to gain more insight into the microbiota-PRR interaction that might help designing medications for various forms of intestinal disorders emanating from disruption of this signaling. In this chapter, the contribution of microbiota to the PRR signaling and responses is discussed. Possible opportunities for employing the microbiota to alleviate gastrointestinal diseases are also highlighted.

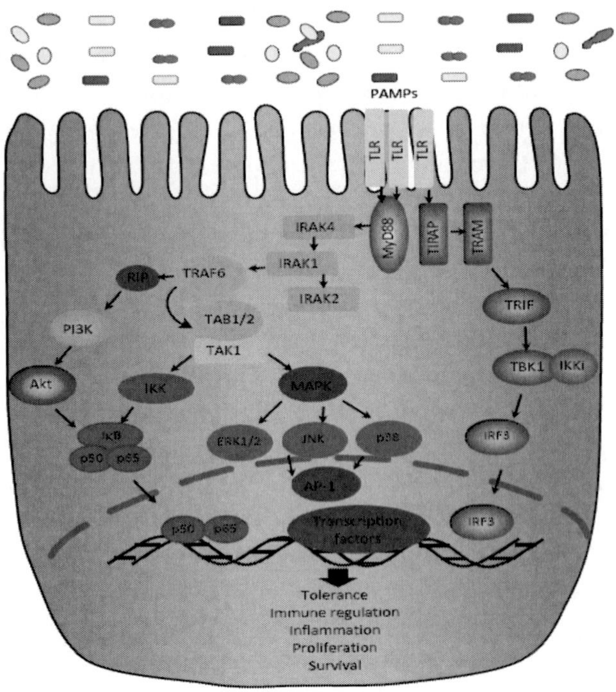

Figure 1. Microbiota-Toll like receptor signaling for intestinal immunity.

Microbiota signaling through TLR in a MyD88-dependent manner activates various intermediate factors that culminate in activation of p50-p65 dimer, ERK1/2, JNK, and p38. The MyD88-independent signaling leads to activation of IRF3. All the activated factors translocate intranuclearly and cause production of mediators for tolerance, immune regulation, inflammation, proliferation, and survival. All these effector products and functions are essential for maintaining intestinal immunity during health and disease. AP, activator protein; ERK, extracellular-regulated kinases; IκB, inhibitory kappa B; IKK, inhibitory kappa B kinase; IRAK, interleukin-1 receptor-associated kinase-like; IRF, interferon regulatory factor; IRF, interferon-regulatory factors; JNK, c-Jun N-terminal kinase activation; MAPK, mitogen activated protein kinase; MyD88, myeloid differentiation primary response gene (88); NF-κB, nuclear factor kappa B; PAMPS, pathogen-associated molecular patterns; RIP, routing information protocol; TAB, TAK1 binding protein; TAK, serine/threonine kinase; TBK, TANK-binding kinase; TIRAP, TIR-domain-containing adaptor protein; TLRs, Toll-like receptors; TRAF, TNF (tumor necrosis factor) receptor-associated factor; TRAM, TRIF related adaptor molecule; TRIF, TIR (Toll/IL-1 receptor) domain-containing adaptor protein inducing interferon-β.

PRRs for Intestinal Innate Immunity

PPR is a primitive part of the immune system that detects microbial antigens and transducer signals. To induce immune responses, commensal microbes are recognized by PRRs, which in turn regulate mucosal innate immunity and inflammatory responses. PRRs are proteins expressed by cells of innate immune system to detect microbe-associated molecular patterns (MAMPs or "infectious non-self") or endogenous "danger signals" derived from stressed, damaged or infected tissue. The detection leads to stimulation of intestinal innate immunity that initiates adaptive immune responses (Schlee 2013). MAMPs include peptidoglycans, lipoproteins, lipopolysaccharides, teichoic acids, CpG DNA motif, double strand RNA and flagellin. They mediate their signals through activation and maturation of antigen presenting cells (APCs) such as DCs (Szabo and Rajnavolgyi 2013).

TLR Signaling

Among PRRs, TLR are the first-discovered and the most well characterized member of PRRs. They are expressed by epithelial cells and APCs (including DCs and macrophages) and are responsible for initial recognition of specific pathogen-associated molecular patterns (PAMPs), discrimination between pathogens and harmless microbes and development of appropriate innate and acquired immune responses (Michelsen and Arditi 2007). They can be located at the cell surface, e.g., TLR1, 2, 4, 5, 6, 10 (Kawai and Akira 2006; Barton and Kagan 2009; Wagner 2012; Kamdar et al., 2013) or intracellularly, e.g., TLR3, 7, 8, 9 (Rakoff-Nahoum and Medzhitov 2008; Wagner 2012; Kamdar et al., 2013). Activation of TLR signaling through recognition of PAMPs leads to dimerization and induction of cell signaling through a series of adaptor molecules such as MyD88, TIR (Toll/IL-1 receptor) domain-containing adaptor protein inducing interferon (IFN)-β (TRIF), interferon regulatory factor (IRF), and TNF receptor-associated factor (TRAF) (Figure 1). This signaling activates NF-κB, activator protein (AP)-1, or IRFs (Kawai and Akira 2006; Rhee 2011). The transactivation of these factors leads to transcriptional activation of genes encoding for pro-inflammatory cytokines, chemokines and co-stimulatory molecules as well as type I interferons, which subsequently control the activation of antigen-specific adaptive immune response (Bermudez-Brito et al., 2014; Song et al., 2014).

Influence of Microbiota on TLR Signaling during Health and Disease

Signaling through TLR co-ligands

The TLR-microbiota interaction modulates immune genes for gut immunity ranging from tolerance to combating pathogens. For instance, TLR2/6 co-ligands prime DCs to become tolerogenic and promote the polarization of IL-10-producing regulatory T cells (Tr1). Furthermore, activation of co-ligands TLR2/1 directs DCs to produce greater amounts of IL-12p40 and low levels of IL-10, thereby promoting the differentiation of Th1 or Th17 cells (DePaolo et al., 2008; DePaolo et al., 2012). The variations in these responses are due to differences in the down-stream effector pathways. Whereas TLR2/1 signals through p38-MAPK, TLR2/6 mediates its effect through c-Jun N-terminal kinase (JNK) activation (Figure 3) (DePaolo et al., 2008).

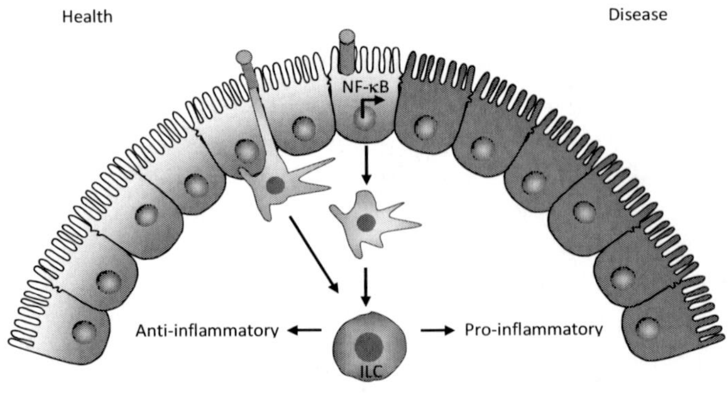

Figure 2. Microbiota-induced activation of innate lymphoid cells through Toll-like receptor signaling.

Commensal bacteria signal through Toll-like receptors found on epithelial and dendritic cells. This signaling activate transcription factors leading to stimulation of lamina propria innate lymphoid cells (ILC) that, depending upon the nature of antigen, induce immune homeostasis (via anti-inflammatory role) or inflammatory reaction during disease. NF-κB, nuclear factor kappa B.

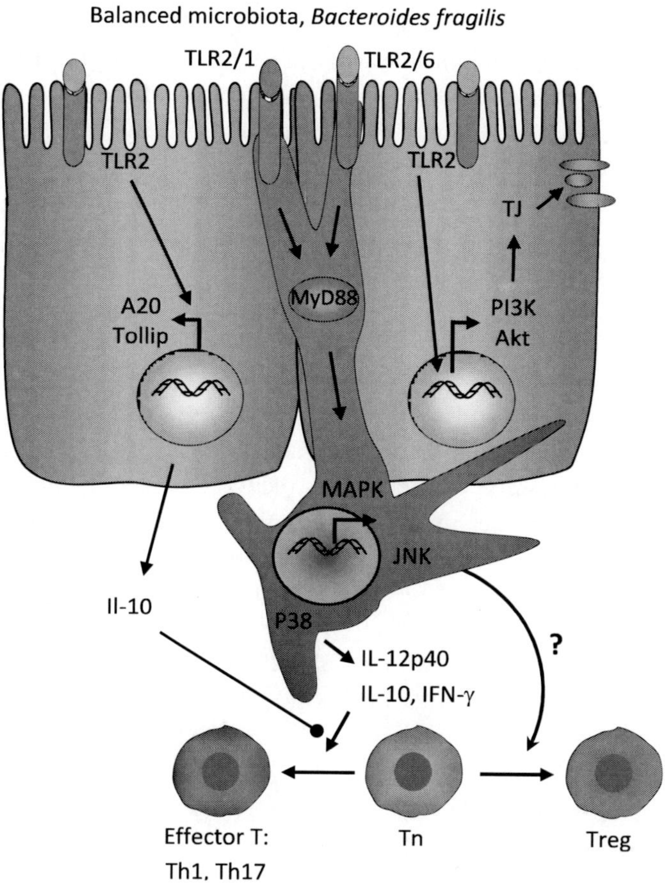

Figure 3. Microbiota-Toll-like receptor interaction in intestinal epithelial and dendritic cells. Balanced microbiota or specific commensal species like *Bacteroides fragilis* are capable of signalling through co-ligands TLR2/1 and TLR2/6 on dendritic cells. The signalling is MyD88-dependent and activates MAPK to drive T cell differentiation and protect the intestine. In addition, the microbiota and *Bacteroides fragilis* protect the intestine by signalling through intestinal epithelial TLR2. This signalling curbs generation of inflammatory effector T cells to prevent inflammation and induces production of tight junction proteins that strengthen the intestinal epithelial barrier integrity to inhibit microbial translocation into the submucosa to cause diseases. IFN, interferon; IL, interleukin; JNK, c-Jun N-terminal kinase; MAPK, mitogen activated protein kinase; Th, T helper cell; TJ, tight junction proteins; TLR, Toll-like receptor; Tn, naïve T cell; Treg, regulatory T cell.

TLR signaling through ligands also benefits microbiota during disease by providing nutrition from within the body. This has recently been reported by Pickard and colleagues (Pickard et al., 2014) who observed that systemic exposure of TLR ligands induces secretion of IL-22 by DCs that activates IECs to express fucosyltransferase 2 leading to α(1,2)-fucosylation of the IECs. The fucosylated proteins are shed into the intestinal lumen to produce fucose that is metabolized by the microbiota during acute disease. In so doing, the microbiota assists in keeping gut immunity during disease-induced stress.

Signaling through TLR1

Literature is scarce about the microbiotal influence on TLR-1 signaling to drive intestinal immunity. Nonetheless, there is evidence that microbiota influences intestinal innate immune functioning through activation of TLR1. Some members of the microbiota, e.g., *Lactobacillus rhamnosus* or their cell-free culture supernatants increase the expression of TLR1 and suppress pro-inflammatory cytokine production by DCs challenged by pathogenic *Escherichia coli* (Bermudez-Brito et al., 2014). The TLR1-mediated anti-inflammatory property is important in curbing impending intestinal disease.

Signaling through TLR2

The microbiotal lipoproteins modulate TLR2 signaling to induce tolerance and prevent inflammation in healthy and diseased gut. This is mediated through increased expression of negative regulators, such as Tollip and A20, and activation of cell signaling pathways that induce production of anti-inflammatory IL-10 (Boone et al., 2004; Cario et al., 2007). The produced IL-10 inhibits macrophage and DC effector functions to limit inflammatory responses (Cario 2008). Alterations in TLR2-mediated NF-κB activation in APCs (such as caspase activation and recruitment domain (CARD15) or NOD-2 mutations), lead to mucosal inflammation through exaggerated IFN-γ, IL-12 and IL-23 production (Figure 3) (Watanabe et al., 2004). A recent study on mechanisms of microbiotal tolerance to the intestinal environment has indicated involvement of dephosphorylation and inactivation of microbiota (symbiont) MAMP lipid A by host alkaline phosphatases (APs). The APs work in synergy with a peptidoglycan recognition protein. The latter inactivates symbiont-exported peptidoglycan monomer to alter the symbiont

MAMPs and promote persistence of the partnership. These activities serve to "tame" MAMPs as well as maintain mutualisms (Rader et al., 2012).

It has been demonstrated that the microbiota *Bacteroides fragilis* through its surface polysaccharide A binds to TLR2 and promotes IL-10 production in $CD4^+$ T cells. In so doing it restrains Th17 responses and enhances its own colonization of the gut (Round et al., 2011). The microbiota translocates into the lumen when T-cell-intrinsic TLR2 signaling is lacking. This translocation could imply strategic colonization to maintain homeostasis. The same mechanism used by *B. fragilis* to colonize host tissue is employed to protect the host from autoimmunity. In this case, the bacterial polysaccharide A signals to T cells through TLR2 and triggers induction of an anti-inflammatory population of regulatory T (Treg) cells within the intestine. The end result is intestinal protection (Lai et al., 2009; Round et al., 2011). Recently, a microbiota member, *Lactobacillus rhamnosus* has shown another ability of the microbiota to enhance innate immunity. This is exhibited by inducing expression of TLR2 gene that suppresses pro-inflammatory cytokine production by DCs challenged by *E. coli* to potentially curb intestinal diseases (Bermudez-Brito et al., 2014).

Another protective PRR signaling through TLR2 involves maintenance of intestinal barrier integrity. Some studies have shown that TLR2 signaling and subsequent activation of TLR2/1 heterodimers by a synthetic triacylated lipoprotein analog Pam_3CysSK_4, maintains tight junction integrity by preserving zonula occludens-1-associated barrier via activation of PI3K and Akt (Rakoff-Nahoum et al., 2004; Cario 2008). This signaling may protect the host against acute mechanical intestinal injury involving tight junctions and diseases due to leaky gut such as inflammatory bowel disease and allergy (Malago 2014).

Signaling through TLR4

Microbiota-TLR4 signaling has also been demonstrated. Signaling through TLR4 alters the gastrointestinal motility (to clear pathogens), maintains commensal populations, induces goblet cell differentiation, overexpresses antimicrobial peptides and inhibits pro-inflmmatory cytokines and impending colitis (Anitha et al., 2012; Sodhi et al., 2012; Bermudez-Brito et al., 2014). This effect occurs following TLR4 stimulation by intraperitoneal LPS that exerts distinct functional effect on the intestinal motility via MyD88-dependent and -independent pathways (Moossavi and Rezaei 2012). It can also be due to the ability of individual microbiota species such as *Lactobacillus rhamnosus* to activate expression of TLR4 gene that leads to suppression of pathogen-induced production of pro-inflammatory cytokines (Figure 4) (Bermudez-Brito et al., 2014).

Furthermore, signaling through TLR4 results in regulation of transcription of α-defensin genes and β-defensin-2 genes in response to alterations in the intestinal microbiota (Vora et al., 2004; Menendez et al., 2013). This regulation restores microbiotal population that subsequently maintains the gut immunity. It has also been shown that disruption of immunity leading to intestinal inflammation such as necrotizing enterocolitis in children and preterm infants occurs following uncontrolled or overexpression of TLR4 by enteric microbes (Gribar et al., 2009; Wolfs et al., 2010). Additionally, enteric disorders can also occur following alterations in microbiota with an increase in proportions of *Bacteroidetes* and less *Firmicutes* (Figure 4).

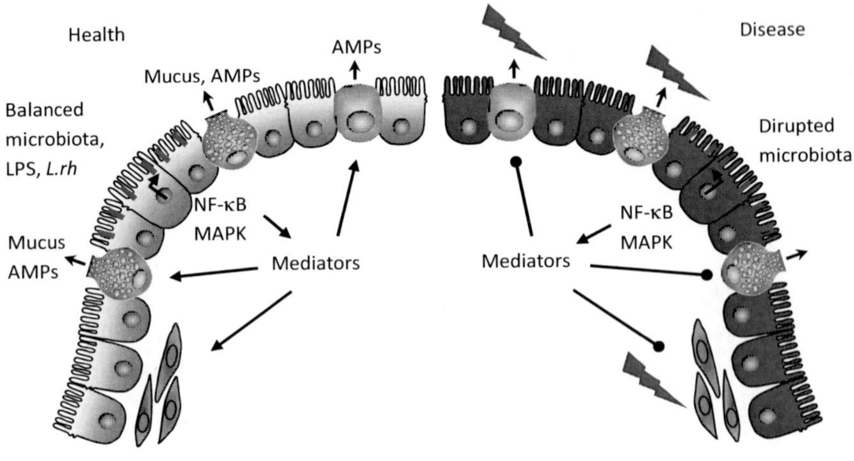

Figure 4. Microbiota signalling through epithelial Toll-like receptors during health and disease. During health, balanced microbiota, microbial lipopolysaccharides and specific commensals like *Lactobacillus rhamnosus* trigger production of protective mediators. The mediators induce production of antimicrobials and mucus as well as control smooth muscle-driven intestinal motility to eliminate pathogens and protect the intestine. Absence or disruption of microbiota generates pro-inflammatory mediators that impair protective functions leading to disease. AMPs, antimicrobial peptides; LPS, lipopolysaccharides; *L.rh*, *Lactobacillus rhamnosus*; MAPK, mitogen activated protein kinase; NF-κB, nuclear factor kappa B.

Such an imbalance leads to activation of TLR signaling, expression of pro-inflammatory cytokines and ulcerative colitis. This colitis is delayed when microbiota signaling through TLR4 is blocked or disrupted (Im et al., 2014; Ren et al., 2014).

Signaling through TLR5

A PRR signaling via TLR5 is depicted by the observation that most of the IEC lines are potently responsive to flagellin, a specific ligand for TLR5 (Rhee et al., 2003; Honko and Mizel 2005) and hyporesponsive to Pam_3Cys and LPS, which are ligands for TLR2 and TLR4, respectively (Abreu et al., 2001; Abreu et al., 2002). TLR5 plays an important role in protection against enterobacterial invasion by producing pro-inflammatory cytokines (Hayashi et al., 2001). As an alternative response to maintain immunity in the absence of TLR5 signaling, TLR5 knock-out (TLR5KO) mice exhibit elevated levels of host defense genes that mediate innate and adaptive immunity in the gut rendering these mice immune to *Salmonella.* Such changes include antimicrobial peptides, serum and fecal immunoglobulin (Ig)A and IgG and transport proteins in the gut (Uematsu et al., 2006; Vijay-Kumar et al., 2008). Other studies have shown that induction of colitis in $TLR5^{-/-}$ mice is associated with significant shifts in the composition of the microbiota (Vijay-Kumar et al., 2007). Transferring the microbiota from these animals into germ-free wild-type mice reproduces the disease (Vijay-Kumar et al., 2007; Caricilli et al., 2011). TLR5 can also influence gut microbiota-derived MAMPs to translocate into the portal circulation and promote hepatic monocyte influx in germ-free mice. In so doing, it shapes liver immunity and Kupffer cell phenotype (Corbitt et al., 2013). This signaling may affect the intestinal immunity.

Signaling through TLR9

The microbiota also mediates its signaling through TLR9 activation. This can occur via basolateral and apical surface domains of TLR9 as well as endosomal response in epithelial cells (Van IJzendoorn et al., 2000; Lee et al., 2006; Yu et al., 2014). The variations in signaling on the apical or basolateral surfaces determine whether the response is tolerogenic or inflammatory, respectively. Apical activation of TLR9, which is directly influenced by luminal microbiota, does not induce activation of the inflammatory NF-κB.

Instead, it induces expression of Frizzled 5, a regulator of Paneth cell maturation, and production of antimicrobial peptides. In addition, according to Yu and colleagues, intestinal host-microbiota homeostasis is controlled by Rab11a, a gene adjacent to Crohn's disease risk locus which is also a recycling endosome resident GTPase. To institute this role, Rab11a maintains a homeostatic intracellular distribution of TLR9 (Yu et al., 2014). Activation of NF-κB and subsequent inflammatory response occur following basolateral stimulation of TLR9 (Lee et al., 2006).

Of recent, Farnesoid X Receptor (FXR), a nuclear receptor and bile acid sensor highly expressed in entero-hepatic tissues that regulates lipid metabolism and innate immunity, has been linked to microbiota role in host's innate immunity. The FXR function and its target gene SHP, a small heterodimer partner, in the intestine is downregulated by membrane TLR2, 4, 5 and 6 and upregulated by intracellular TLR3, 7, 8 and 9. This effect is TLR9- and MyD88-dependent but TNF-α independent. Intestinal inflammation induced in mice by trinitrobenzene sulphonic acid (TNBS) downregulates the intestinal expression of FXR and protection against TNBS colitis by CpG, a TLR-9 ligand. This effect is lost in $FXR^{-/-}$ mice. Further, activation of FXR protects $TLR9^{-/-}$ and $MyD88^{-/-}$ mice from colitis. These effects involve IRF7 recruitment (Renga et al., 2013). The role of microbiota on chemical colitis has also been demonstrated by other researchers. Negishi and others (Negishi et al., 2012) reported that IRF3, activated by microbiota-derived nucleic acids (Figure 1), is critical for the suppression of dextran sulfate sodium (DSS)-induced colitis as IRF3-deficient mice exhibit lethal defects of the colitis, accompanied by marked defects in the gene induction for thymic stromal lymphopoietin (TSLP). TSLP is a cytokine essential for protection of the large intestine and IRF3 activates the gene promoter of TSLP via IRF-binding sequences.

Microbiota signaling through TLR9 is partly due to recognition of unmethylated CpG motifs in microbial DNA by the TLR9. GTCGTT is an optimal motif that stimulates TLR9 signaling. Beneficial bacteria belonging to *Proteobacteria*, *Bacteroidetes* and *Actinobacteria* (e.g., bifidobacteria) and individual species like *Enterococcus faecalis*, *Lactobacillus casei*, *Lactobacillus plantarum* and *Lactobacillus rhamnosus*, contain high counts of GTCGTT motifs. The high number, coupled with adequate level of TLR9 stimulation drives an optimal microbiota function to maintain intestinal immunity. This could prevent allergy and autoimmune diseases by controlling Th1/Th2 balance (Kant et al., 2013).

Signaling through IRAK-M

Maintenance of intestinal innate and adaptive immunity by microbiota can also be mediated by a member of IL-1 receptor-associated kinase (IRAK) family IRAK-M, mainly expressed on macrophages and mononuclear cells. IRAK-M negatively regulates TLR signaling through inhibition of MyD88, the adaptor molecule downstream all TLRs except TLR3 (Figure 1). Deficiency of IRAK-M enhances NF-κB activity and expression of inflammatory cytokines in response to several TLR ligands. This molecule is critical in innate immunity functioning for anti-pathogen responses, inflammation and autoimmunity. It has recently been reported that antibiotically altered gut microbiota promotes colitis associated cancer in mice deficient of IRAK-M (Klimesova et al., 2013). Treatment of wild-type mice by antibiotics lowers the numbers of Treg cells in colon, alters the gut microbiota composition, and decreases β-glucuronidase activity. However, the β-glucuronidase activity is not as low as in germ-free mice and the treatment reduces the incidence and severity of tumors. On the contrary, IRAK-M-deficient mice treated with antibiotics develop invasive tumors, cannot be rescued from severe carcinogenesis phenotype by the decrease in β-glucuronidase activity, and have increased levels of pro-inflammatory cytokines in the tumor tissue (Klimesova et al., 2013).

Signaling through IEC Circadian Clock

A recent study by Mukherji and others (Mukherji et al., 2013) has revealed that the integrity of IECs circadian clock is required for microbiota-IECs dialog. They observed that the antiphasic expression of the retinoic acid-related orphan receptor (ROR)-α activator and RevErbα repressor clock output regulators in the IECs generates a circadian rhythmic TLR expression. The expression converts the temporally arrhythmic microbiota signaling into circadian rhythmic JNK and inhibitory kappa B kinase (IKK)-β activities. This signaling prevents RevErbα activation by PPARα that would disrupt the circadian clock. In addition, the JNK and IKK-β activities, together with RORα and RevErbα, enable timing homeostatic functions of numerous genes with IECs circadian events through activation of AP-1 and NF-κB. Deficiency of the microbiota signaling induces a prediabetic syndrome due to ileal corticosterone overproduction consequent to clock disruption.

NLR SIGNALING

Apart from the TLR, other PRR employed by IECs are the NOD-1 and 2 proteins signaling from NLR. NOD-1 and 2 are leucine-rich repeat (LRR) intracellular proteins and sensors of viral and bacterial products in the induction of inflammatory responses (Franchi et al., 2009; Langefeld et al., 2009). The bacterial sensed molecules include products of synthesis, degradation and remodelling of peptidoglycan. NOD-1 recognizes products containing γ-D-glutamyl-mesodiaminopimelic acid of Gram-negative bacteria while NOD-2 reacts with bacterial cell wall component muramyl dipeptide (MDP) of most bacteria (Girardin et al., 2003; Inohara et al., 2003; Strober et al., 2006). The NOD-2 signaling is most likely mediated by direct ligand binding of MDP to the LRR domain of NOD-2 (Figure 5) (Mo et al., 2012). The end result of signaling by both NOD-1 and 2 is activation of the transcription factor NF-κB and its subsequent inflammatory response (Ogura et al., 2001; Tig and Davis 2005).

The NLR family is composed of various subfamilies based on N-terminus motifs. They include CARD also called NOD subfamily, PYRIN domain protein also called NALP (NACHT-LRR-PYD-containing proteins) subfamily and baculoviral inhibitor-of-apoptosis protein repeat (BIR) domain, also called neuronal apoptosis inhibitory protein (NAIP) subfamily (Tig and Davis 2005; Fritz et al., 2006; Meylan et al., 2006). CARD mediates NOD-2-dependent NF-κB activation upon recruitment of receptor interacting protein kinase 2 (RIPK2), which binds to NOD-2 through homotypic CARD–CARD interactions (Ogura et al., 2001; Voss et al., 2006). Both NALP and NAIP subfamilies form part of multiprotein complexes called the inflammasomes that activate several caspases including 1, 4, and 5 following damage-associated molecular pattern molecules (DAMPs) recognition (Figure 5). The activation of caspases leads to cleavage of the proforms of IL-1-like cytokines IL-1β, IL-18 and IL-33 into their active forms and subsequent inflammatory response (Martinon et al., 2002; Martinon and Tschopp 2004; Strowig et al., 2012).

Influence of Microbiota on NLR Signaling

Although fewer studies have focused on microbiota-NOD interaction than on TLR, there is enough evidence on this crosstalk and the resulting enhanced intestinal immunity. For instance in mice infected with pathogenic

Streptococcus pneumoniae and *Staphylococcus aureus*, NOD-1 recognizes microbiotal peptidoglycan and primes systemic innate immunity by enhancing the cytotoxicity of bone-marrow derived neutrophils in response to the systemic infection (Clarke et al., 2010). Some studies have shown involvement of NOD-1 and 2 in production of antimicrobial peptides following PRR engagement by microbiotal ligands. The signaling activates Paneth cells that increase their production of antimicrobial peptides in response to abnormally high bacterial counts. It can be mediated via the MyD88-dependent TLR (Vaishnava et al., 2008) or NOD-1 and 2 activation (Voss et al., 2006). The produced antimicrobial peptides impede translocation and dissemination of microbes across the mucosal barrier (Vaishnava et al., 2008).

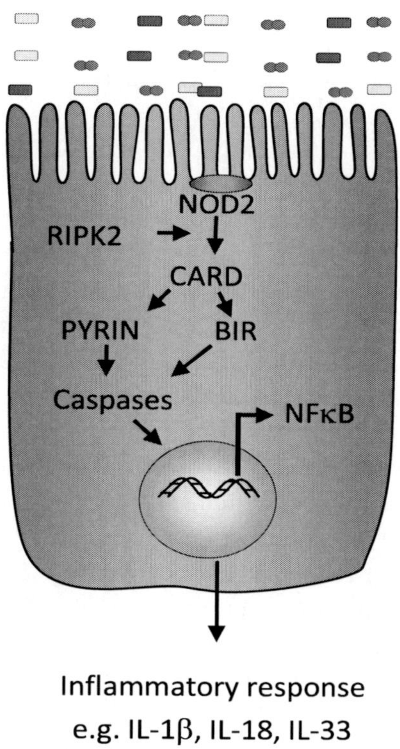

Figure 5. Microbiota signalling through intestinal epithelial NOD-like receptors. By signalling through NOD2 receptors, several molecules are involved before activation of transcription factors. The microbiota-NOD2-induced gene activation culminates in production of inflammatory mediators that curb intestinal diseases and maintain immunity. NOD, nucleotide oligomerization domain.

NLR Signaling and Intestinal Diseases

The significance of NLR signaling is vivid in intestinal diseases like Crohn’s disease. NOD-2 was the first gene associated with susceptibility to this disease (Hugot et al., 2001). Patients with Crohn's disease have NOD-2 mutations which suppress activation of NF-κB. Researchers have proposed diminished production of defensin by Paneth cells and lower cytoprotective function at the epithelial layer to contribute to the condition. Another proposed possibility is the failure of the NOD-2 mutated variants expressed in Crohn’s patients to activate the TLR2 signaling, since NOD-2 activation inhibits TLR2 signaling (Xavier and Podolsky 2007).

CONCLUSION

Both TLR and NLR are important drivers of microbiotal function on innate immune response. Most intestinal microbes signal through PRR. In turn the PRR highly discriminates variations in antigens and subsequently trigger tightly regulated and focused response to a particular antigen. Owing to millions of luminal antigens, the PRR discriminative ability and signaling are extraordinarily efficient and essential to gut innate immunity. Microbiotal dysbiosis significantly impairs this signaling leading to diseases. Such diseases result from pro-inflammatory responses generated by transcription factors activated by antigens from disrupted microbiota. They can also come from enteral pathogens. Restoration of disrupted microbiota to normality drives anti-inflammatory responses, ameliorates the diseases, and protects the intestine. Currently the microbiota-PRR protective signaling has not been employed in this respect. However, the potential can be exploited to develop therapeutics that will improve microbiota profile, diversity and protective influence on PRR signaling. This can be achieved through research employing modern technology like genomics that are capable of exploring the influence of microbiota to PRR signaling at the level of specific bacterial species. Such approach should be a focus of future research.

REFERENCES

Abreu, MT; Arnold, ET; Thomas, LS; et al. TLR4 and MD-2 expression is regulated by immune-mediated signals in human intestinal epithelial cells. *J Biol Chem.*, 2002, 277, 20431-20437.

Abreu, MT; Vora, P; Faure, E; et al. Decreased expression of Toll-like receptor-4 and MD-2 correlates with intestinal epithelial cell protection against dysregulated proinflammatory gene expression in response to bacterial lipopolysaccharide. *J Immunol.*, 2001, 167, 1609-1616.

Anitha, M; Vijay-Kumar, M; Sitaraman, SV; et al. Gut microbial products regulate murine gastrointestinal motility via Toll-like receptor 4 signaling. *Gastroenterology*, 2012, 143, 1006-1016.

Barton, GM; Kagan, JC. A cell biological view of Toll-like receptor function: regulation through compartmentalization. *Nat Rev Immunol.*, 2009, 9, 535-542.

Bermudez-Brito, M; Muñoz-Quezada, S; Gomez-Llorente, C; et al. Lactobacillus rhamnosus and its cell-free culture supernatant differentially modulate inflammatory biomarkers in Escherichia coli-challenged human dendritic cells. *Br J Nutr.*, 2014, 111, 1727-1737.

Boone, DL; Turer, EE; Lee, EG; et al. The ubiquitin-modifying enzyme A20 is required for termination of Toll-like receptor responses. *Nat Immunol.*, 2004, 5, 1052-1060.

Caricilli, AM; Picardi, PK; de, Abreu, LL; et al. Gut microbiota is a key modulator of insulin resistance in TLR 2 knockout mice. *PLoS Biol.*, 2011, 9, e1001212.

Cario E Barrier-protective function of intestinal epithelial Toll-like receptor 2. Mucosal Immunonol., 2008, 1, S62-S66.

Cario, E; Gerken, G; Podolsky, DK. Toll-like receptor 2 controls mucosal inflammation by regulating epithelial barrier function. *Gastroenterology.*, 2007, 132, 1359-1374.

Clarke, TB; Davis, KM; Lysenko, ES; et al. Recognition of peptidoglycan from the microbiota by Nod1 enhances systemic innate immunity. *Nat Med.*, 2010, 16, 228–231.

Corbitt, N; Kimura, S; Isse, K; et al. Gut bacteria drive Kuppfer cell expansion via MAMP-mediated ICAM-1 induction on sinusoidal endothelium and influence preservation-reperfusion injury after orthotopic liver transplantation. *Am J Pathol.*, 2013, 182, 180-191.

DePaolo, RW; Kamdar, K; Khakpour, S; et al. A specific role for TLR1 in protective T(H)17 immunity during mucosal infection. *J Exp Med.*, 2012, 209, 1437-1444.

DePaolo, RW; Tang, F; Kim, I; et al. Toll-like receptor 6 drives differentiation of tolerogenic dendritic cells and contributes to LcrV-mediated plague pathogenesis. *Cell Host Microbe.*, 2008, 4, 350-361.

Franchi, L; Warner, N; Viani, K; et al. Function of Nod-like receptors in microbial recognition and host defense. *Immunol Rev.*, 2009, 277, 106-128.

Fritz, JH; Ferrero, RL; Philpott, DJ; et al. Nod-like proteins in immunity, inflammation and disease. *Nat Immunol.*, 2006, 7, 1250-1257.

Girardin, SE; Boneca, IG; Viala, J; et al. Nod2 is a general sensor of peptidoglycan through muramyl dipeptide (MDP) detection. *J Biol Chem.*, 2003, 278, 8869–8872.

Gribar, SC; Sodhi, CP; Richardson, WM; et al. Reciprocal expression and signaling of TLR4 and TLR9 in the pathogenesis and treatment of necrotizing enterocolitis. *J Immunol.*, 2009, 182, 636-646.

Hayashi, F; Smith, KD; Ozinsky, A; et al. The innate immune response to bacterial flagellin is mediated by Toll-like receptor 5. *Nature.*, 2001, 410, 1099-1103.

Honko, AN; Mizel, SB. Effects of flagellin on innate and adaptive immunity. *Immunol Res.*, 2005, 33, 83-101.

Hugot, JP; Chamaillard, M; Zouali, H; et al. Association of NOD2 leucine-rich repeat variants with susceptibility to Crohn's disease. *Nature.* 2001, 411, 599-603.

Im, E; Jung, J; Pothoulakis, C; et al. Disruption of Pten speeds onset and increases severity of spontaneous colitis in IL-10($^{-/-}$) mice. *Gastroenterology.*, 2014, 147, 667-679.

Inohara, N; Ogura, Y; Fontalba, A; et al. Host recognition of bacterial muramyl dipeptide mediated through NOD2. Implications for Crohn’s disease. *J Biol Chem.*, 2003, 278, 5509-5512.

Jeannin, P; Jaillon, S; Delneste, Y. Pattern recognition receptors in the immune response against dying cells. *Curr Opin Immunol.*, 2008 Oct,20(5), 530-7.

Kamdar, K; Nguyen, V; DePaolo, RW. Toll-like receptor signaling and regulation of intestinal immunity. *Virulence.*, 2013, 4, 207-212.

Kant, R; de Vos, WM; Palva, A; et al. Immunostimulatory CpG motifs in the genomes of gut bacteria and their role in human health and disease. *J Med Microbiol.*, 2014, 63(Pt 2), 293-308.

Kawai, T; Akira, S. TLR signaling. *Cell Death Differ.*, 2006, 13, 816-825

Klimesova, K; Kverka, M; Zakostelska, Z, et al. Altered gut microbiota promotes colitis-associated cancer in IL-1 receptor-associated kinase M-deficient mice. *Inflamm Bowel Dis.*, 2013, 19, 1266-1277.

Lai, Y; Di, Nardo, A; Nakatsuji, T; et al. Commensal bacteria regulate Toll-like receptor 3-dependent inflammation after skin injury. *Nat Med.*, 2009, 15, 1377–1382.

Langefeld, T; Mohamed, W; Ghai, R; et al. Toll-like receptors and NOD-like receptors: domain architecture and cellular signaling. *Adv Exp Med Biol.*, 2009, 653, 48-57.

Lee, J; Mo, JH; Katakura, K; et al. Maintenance of colonic homeostasis by distinctive apical TLR9 signaling in intestinal epithelial cells. *Nat Cell Biol.*, 2006, 8, 1327-1336.

Malago, JJ. Contribution of microbiota to the intestinal physicochemical barrier. *Benef Microbes.*, 2014, In Press.

Malago, JJ; Koninkx, JF; van, Dijk, JE. The heat shock response and cytoprotection of the intestinal epithelium. *Cell Stress Chaperones.*, 2002, 7, 191-199.

Martinon, F; Burns, K; Tschopp, J. The inflammasome: a molecular platform triggering activation of inflammatory caspases and processing of proIL-beta. *Mol Cell.*, 2002, 10, 417–426.

Martinon, F; Tschopp, J. Inflammatory caspases: linking an intracellular innate immune system to autoinflammatory diseases. *Cell.*, 2004, 117, 561-574.

Menendez, A; Willing, BP; Montero, M; et al. Bacterial stimulation of the TLR-MyD88 pathway modulates the homeostatic expression of ileal paneth cell α-defensins. *J Innate Immun.*, 2013, 5, 39-49.

Meylan, E; Tschopp, J; Karin, M. Intracellular pattern recognition receptors in the host response. *Nature.*, 2006, 442, 39-44.

Michelsen, KS; Arditi, M. Toll-like receptors and innate immunity in gut homeostasis and pathology. *Curr Opin Hematol.*, 2007, 14, 48–54.

Mo, J; Boyle, JP; Howard, CB, et al. Pathogen sensing by nucleotide-binding oligomerization domain-containing protein 2 (NOD2) is mediated by direct binding to muramyl dipeptide and ATP. *J Biol Chem.*, 2012, 287, 23057–23067.

Moossavi, S; Rezaei, N. Host-microbiota interaction is MyD88-independent in the intestinal tract under physiologic condition. *Avicenna J Med Biotechnol.*, 2012, 4, 210-211.

Mukherji, A; Kobiita, A; Ye, T; et al. Homeostasis in intestinal epithelium is orchestrated by the circadian clock and microbiota cues transduced by TLRs. *Cell.*, 2013, 153, 812-827.

Negishi, H; Miki, S; Sarashina, H; et al. Essential contribution of IRF3 to intestinal homeostasis and microbiota-mediated Tslp gene induction. *Proc Natl Acad Sci USA.*, 2012, 109, 21016-21021.

Ogura, Y; Inohara, N; Benito, A; et al. Nod2, a Nod1/Apaf-1 family member that is restricted to monocytes and activates NF-kappaB. *J Biol Chem.*, 2001, 276, 4812–4818.

Pickard, JM; Maurice, CF; Kinnebrew, MA; et al. Rapid fucosylation of intestinal epithelium sustains host-commensal symbiosis in sickness. *Nature.*, 2014, In Press

Rader, BA; Kremer, N; Apicella, MA; et al. Modulation of symbiont lipid A signaling by host alkaline phosphatases in the squid-vibrio symbiosis. *mBio.*, 2012, 3, e00093.

Rakoff-Nahoum, S; Medzhitov, R. Innate immune recognition of the indigenous microbial flora. *Mucosal Immunol.*, 2008, 1 Suppl 1, S10-14.

Rakoff-Nahoum, S; Paglino, J; Eslami-Varzaneh, F; et al. Recognition of commensal microflora by toll-like receptors is required for intestinal homeostasis. *Cell.*, 2004, 118, 229–241.

Ren, W; Chen, S; Yin, J; et al. Dietary arginine supplementation of mice alters the microbial population and activates intestinal innate immunity. *J Nutr.*, 2014, 144, 988-995.

Renga, B; Mencarelli, A; Cipriani, S; et al. The bile acid sensor FXR is required for immune-regulatory activities of TLR-9 in intestinal inflammation. *PLoS One.*, 2013, 8, e54472.

Rhee, SH. Basic and translational understandings of microbial recognition by Toll-like receptors in the intestine. *J Neurogastroenterol Motil.*, 2011, 17, 28-34.

Rhee, SH; Jones, BW; Toshchakov, V; et al. Toll-like receptors 2 and 4 activate STAT1 serine phosphorylation by distinct mechanisms in macrophages. *J Biol Chem.*, 2003, 278, 22506-22512.

Round, JL; Lee, Sm; Li, J; et al. The Toll-like receptor 2 pathway establishes colonization by a commensal of the human microbiota. *Science.*, 2011, 332, 974–977.

Schenten, D; Medzhitov, R. The control of adaptive immune responses by the innate immune system. *Adv Immunol.*, 2011, 109, 87-124.

Schlee, M. Master sensors of pathogenic RNA - RIG-I like receptors. *Immunobiology.*, 2013, 218, 1322-1235.

Sodhi, CP; Neal, MD; Siggers, R; et al. Intestinal epithelial Toll-like receptor 4 regulates goblet cell development and is required for necrotizing enterocolitis in mice. *Gastroenterology*, 2012, 143, 708-718.

Song, X; Gao, H; Lin, Y; et al. Alterations in the microbiota drive interleukin-17C production from intestinal epithelial cells to promote tumorigenesis. *Immunity.*, 2014, 40, 140-152

Strober, W; Murray, P; Kitani, A; et al. Signaling pathways and molecular interactions of NOD1 and NOD2. *Nat Rev Immunol.*, 2006, 6, 9-20.

Strowig, T; Henao-Mejia, J; Elinav, E; et al. Inflammasomes in health and disease. *Nature.*, 2012, 481, 278–286.

Szabo, A; Rajnavolgyi, E. Collaboration of Toll-like and RIG-I-like receptors in human dendritic cells: tRIGgering antiviral innate immune responses. *Am J Clin Exp Immunol.*, 2013, 2, 195-207.

Tig, JP; Davis, BK. CATERPILLER: a novel gene family important in immunity, cell death, and diseases. *Annu Rev Immunol.*, 2005, 23, 387-414.

Uematsu, S; Jang, MH; Chevrier, N; et al. Detection of pathogenic intestinal bacteria by Toll-like receptor 5 on intestinal CD11c+ lamina propria cells. *Nat Immunol.*, 2006, 7, 868-874.

Vaishnava, S; Behrendt, CL; Ismail, AS; et al. Paneth cells directly sense gut commensals and maintain homeostasis at the intestinal host-microbial interface. *Proc Natl Acad Sci USA.*, 2008, 105, 20858-20863.

Van, IJzendoorn, SC; Maier, O; Van Der Wouden, JM; et al. The subapical compartment and its role in intracellular trafficking and cell polarity. *J Cell Physiol.*, 2000, 184, 151-160.

Vijay-Kumar, M; Aitken, JD; Kumar, A; et al. Toll-like receptor 5-deficient mice have dysregulated intestinal gene expression and nonspecific resistance to Salmonella-induced typhoid-like disease. *Infect Immun.*, 2008, 76, 1276-1281.

Vijay-Kumar, M; Sanders, CJ; Taylor, RT; et al. Deletion of TLR5 results in spontaneous colitis in mice. *J Clin Invest.*, 2007, 117, 3909–3921.

Vora, P; Youdim, A; Thomas, LS; et al. Beta-defensin-2 expression is regulated by TLR signaling in intestinal epithelial cells. *J Immmunol.*, 2004, 173, 5398-5405.

Voss, RH; Kuball, J; Engel, R; et al. Redirection of T cells by delivering a transgenic mouse-derived MDM2 tumor antigen-specific TCR and its humanized derivative is governed by the CD8 coreceptor and affects natural human TCR expression. *Immunol Res.*, 2006, 34, 67-87.

Wagner, H. Toll-like receptors in gastrointestinal diseases. *Dig Dis.*, 2012, 30 Suppl 1, 74-77.

Watanabe, T; Kitani, A; Murray, PJ; et al. NOD2 is a negative regulator of Toll-like receptor 2-mediated T helper type 1 responses. *Nat Immunol.*, 2004, 5, 800-808.

Wolfs, TG; Derikx, JP; Hodin, CM; et al. Localization of the lipopolysaccharide recognition complex in the human healthy and inflamed premature and adult gut. *Inflamm Bowel Dis.*, 2010, 16, 68-75.

Xavier, RJ; Podolsky, DK. Unravelling the pathogenesis of inflammatory bowel disease. *Nature.*, 2007, 448, 427-434

Xue, LY; Ouyang, Q; Zhou, XG; et al. Bacterial immune interaction in experimental colitis. *J Dig Dis.*, 2013, 14, 526-535.

Yu, S; Nie, Y; Knowles, B; et al. TLR sorting by Rab11 endosomes maintains intestinal epithelial-microbial homeostasis. *EMBO J.*, 2014, 33, 1882-1895

Zhong, J; Kyriakis, JM. Dissection of a signaling pathway by which pathogen-associated molecular patterns recruit the JNK and p38 MAPKs and trigger cytokine release. *J Biol Chem.*, 2007, 282, 24246-24254.

Chapter 2

ROLE OF MICROBIOTA TO LEUKOCYTES ENGENDERING INTESTINAL INNATE IMMUNE RESPONSE

ABSTRACT

Leukocytes involved in innate immune system encounter diverse agents ranging from harmless commensal and food proteins to life threatening pathogens, toxins, and other chemical compounds. While these leukocytes are insensitive to harmless agents in terms of inciting inflammatory response, they respond to noxious agents by immediately destroying and eliminating them from the body. This is done through phagocytosis, granulocytosis, degranulation to release enzymes and inflammatory mediators, antigen presentation, and activation of adaptive immune system. These functions are influenced by microbiota whose disruption impairs the optimal functioning of innate immune leukocytes and predisposes the intestine to diseases like allergy, inflammatory bowel diseases, and irritable bowel syndrome. Maneuvers that restore disrupted microbiota benefit patients with these diseases. The current chapter discusses contribution of microbiota to the functioning of killer cells, mast cells, eosinophils, basophils and neutrophils that constitute innate immune cells, focusing on the regulation of their functions during health and disease.

INTRODUCTION

The gut innate immunity provides immediate, non-specific and short lasting defense against infection. It comprises physical barrier, cells in blood and tissues, soluble mediators and mechanisms that defend the host from infection by other organisms in a generic manner. Specifically, it recruits immune cells to sites of infection, activates complement cascade, identifies and removes foreign substances from the body, presents antigens to adaptive immune system to activate it, and acts as a physical barrier against pathogens (Prussin and Metcalfe 2003; Nakanishi 2010; Malago 2014). As pathogens strive to enter the body and cause disease, the innate immune system works as a first line of defense to prevent their entry or eliminate invading pathogens that would otherwise damage the host.

Cells of the innate immune system are mainly leukocytes that include natural killer (NK) cells, mast cells, eosinophils, basophils and the phagocytic cells including macrophages, neutrophils and dendritic cells (DCs). Their functions involve identifying and eliminating antigens and pathogens that might cause disease. Intestinal luminal antigens must activate these cells to cause inflammation which is subsequently promoted and maintained through stimulation of the adaptive immune response. To carry out their functions, these cells are equipped with all necessary ability to combat the microorganisms including expression of receptors, secretion of inflammatory mediators like cytokines, histamine, heparin, proteolytic enzymes, reactive oxygen species, eicosanoids, and growth factors (Horiuchi and Weller 1997; Banderira-Melo et al., 2002; Hofman et al., 2000; Nadeau et al., 2002; Saito et al., 2004; Kato et al., 2005; Hogan et al., 2008; Smith et al., 2012; Bhatnagar et al., 2014; Noti et al., 2014) As they execute their functions, they initiate inflammation by secreting these mediators and antimicrobial agents leading to phagocytosis of microbes and infected cells, antigen presentation, and activation of the adaptive immune system (Hofman et al., 2000; Nadeau et al., 2002; Segal 2005; Nakanishi et al., 2010; Smith et al., 2012; Noti et al., 2014).

The intestinal environment is enriched with diverse commensal microbes and oftentimes challenged by pathogens. While the pathogenic microbes are recognized and selectively eliminated from the body by the cells of the immune system, commensal microbes contribute significantly to supporting the immune system fight the pathogens. Disturbances to the microbiota may fail this support and could lead to diseases like colitis (e.g., chemical, spontaneous, and that occurring in inflammatory bowel disease, IBD), irritable bowel syndrome (IBS), cytomegalovirus, and allergy. Interventions aimed at restoring microbiota profile often ameliorate in part or complete the severity of these diseases. The mechanisms involved in this amelioration involve improvement in the functioning of cells of the innate immune system (Ouwehand et al., 2009; Barbara et al., 2011; Ganal et al., 2012; Gopalakrishnan et al., 2012; Wang et al., 2013; Brenner et al., 2014; Kobayashi et al., 2014). Thus, the influence of microbiota to these cells is fairly evident. Amongst others, the microbiota plays role in regulation of granulocytosis, neutrophil phagocytosis, degranulation and homeostasis, and host resistance to conditions caused by disruption of leukocytes (Deshmukh et al., 2014; Knoop et al., 2014). Gaining insight into the microbiota-innate immune cell interaction could be a prelude towards designing successful therapeutics against disorders caused by abnormalities in this relationship. This chapter describes the contribution of microbiota to the functioning of cells of the gut innate immune system during health and disease.

NK Cells and Innate Lymphoid Cells

NK cells are subsets of granular lymphocytes capable of destroying foreign and dysfunctional cells through degranulation and cell lysis mediated by NK cell-derived interferon (IFN)-γ production (Klose et al., 2013). They belong to innate lymphoid cells (ILCs), some of which are analogous to T helper (Th) cells while others to cytotoxic NK cells. ILCs regulate immune homeostasis and inflammation and play role in gut immunity. Current knowledge categorizes ILCs into three groups (Figure 1). Group 1 ILCs produce type 1 cytokines (i.e., IFN-γ and tumor necrosis factor (TNF)) and comprise ILC1s and NK cells (Spits and Di Santo 2011); group 2 ILCs produce type 2 cytokines (i.e., interleukin (IL)-4, IL-5, IL-9, IL-13) and express transcription factor retinoic acid orphan receptor (ROR)-α and GATA binding protein 3 (GATA3) (Neill et al., 2010); group 3 ILCs produce IL-17A and /or IL-22 and comprise ILC3s and lymphoid tissue-inducer (LTi) cells (Withers et al., 2012). Like other ILCs, NK cells lack a B or T cell receptor and thus do not respond in an antigen-specific manner (Walker et al., 2013). Instead, they recognize their subjects in the absence of antibodies and major histocompatibility class (MHC). The term “natural killer” stems from the idea that they do not require activation to kill cells that lack “self” markers of MHCI (Vivier et al., 2011). This role is so critical because harmful cells lacking MHC1 markers are neither detected nor destroyed by T or other immune cells.

NK cells express several activating receptors including CD16 (FcγRIII) that binds immunoglobulin (Ig)G during antibody-dependent cellular cytotoxicity (Bhatnagar et al., 2014), C-type lectin family receptors like CD94:NKG2 heterodimers for non-classical MHCI molecules (e.g., HLA-E) (Campos et al., 2014) and Ly49 for classical MHCI (Tu et al., 2014), and natural cytotoxic receptors (NCR) for NK killing and release of IFN-γ (Klose et al., 2013). They also express inhibitory receptors like killer-cell immunoglobulin-like receptor (KIR) for both classical and non-classical MHCI, leukocyte inhibitory receptor (LIR or ILT) and Ly49 for classical MHCI (Heidenreich et al., 2012; Kruse et al., 2014)

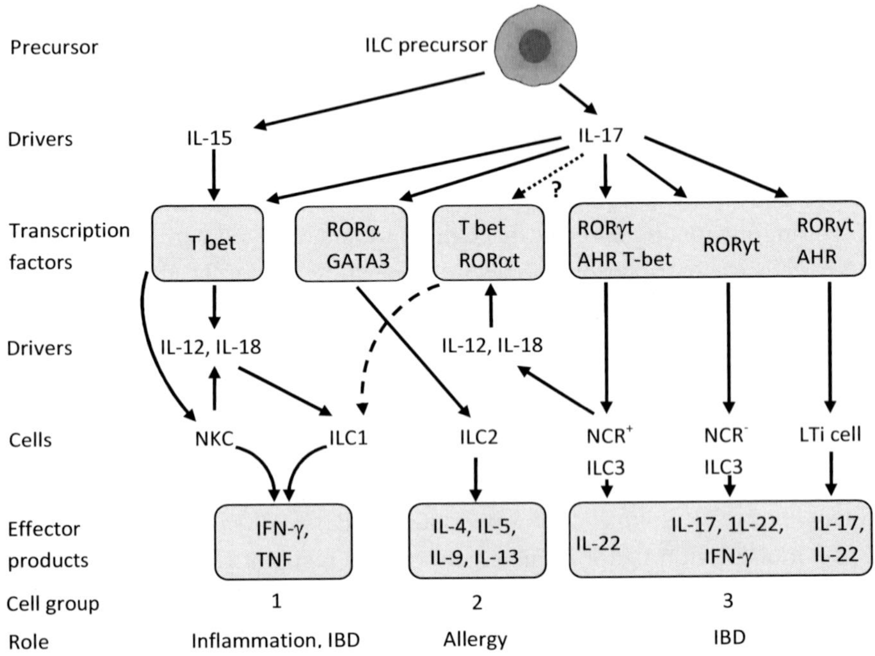

Figure 1. Groups of innate lymphoid cells. Three groups of ILCs i.e., group 1, 2 and 3, are derived from a common precursor exhibiting activation of various transcription factors. The cells are categorised based on their effector products which may determine variations in disease development. AHR, aryl hydrocarbon receptor; IBD, inflammatory bowel disease; IFN, interferon; IL, interleukin; ILC, innate lymphoid cell; LTi, lymphoid tissue-inducer; NCR, natural cytotoxic receptors; NKC, natural killer cell; ROR, retinoic acid orphan receptor; TNF, tumour necrosis factor.

Influence of Microbiota to ILCs

The intestinal microbiota regulates expression of NK cell ligands on intestinal epithelial cells (IECs) to influence NK cell responses. In this regard, it decreases the expression magnitude of NK group 2 member D (NKG2D) ligands on IECs. Absence of microbiota in germ-free and ampicillin-treated mice increases the NKG2D ligand expression while propagation of *Akkermansia muciniphila* by vancomycin which reduces the level of IFN-γ and IL-15, decreases the NKG2D ligand expression. Similarly, dietary xylooligosaccharides-induced increase in *A. muciniphila* decreases the expression of NKG2D ligand while IL-10 deficiency increases NKG2D ligand expression (Hansen et al., 2013).

The necessity of microbiota to mediate NK immune response is further exemplified in germ-free mice in which mononuclear phagocytes residing in nonmucosal lymphoid organs fail to induce inflammatory response genes. This is because the lack of microbiota in germ-free mice severely compromises NK cell priming and immunity despite of normal pattern recognition receptor (PRR) signaling and nuclear translocation of the transcription factors nuclear factor κB and interferon regulatory transcription factor (IRF)3. The lack of microbiota leads to defected binding of these transcription factors to their respective cytokine promoters caused by absence of activating histone marks. Induction of changes at chromatin level by colonizing microbiota poises expression of central inflammatory genes to initiate a powerful systemic immune response (Ganal et al., 2012).

The microbiota promotes a crosstalk between macrophages and ILCs that leads to immune homeostasis in the intestine. This occurs when macrophages sense microbial signals and produce IL-1β that drives RORγt^{+} ILCs to produce granulocyte-macrophage colony-stimulating factor (GM-CSF) that maintains intestinal immune homeostasis (Figure 2). Deficient GM-CSF production alters mononuclear phagocyte effector functions resulting in reduced regulatory T (Treg) cell numbers and impaired oral tolerance (Mortha et al., 2014). Additionally, ILCs, particularly ILC3s, are activated by DCs and IECs to produce IL-22 which triggers production of antimicrobial peptides and defensins. In so doing, ILC3s contribute to maintenance of intestinal homeostasis. Malfunction of ILCs contributes to the development of IBD (Walker et al., 2013). Intestinal immune homeostasis can also be maintained through NFIL3, a transcription factor that regulates multiple immunologic functions including repressing IL-12p40 transcription. It is also a susceptible gene for IBD independent of IL-10 regulation. Myeloid cells respond to IL-10 to express NFIL3. The microbiota activates the NFIL3 to downregulate IL-12p40 and maintains homeostaisis independent of IL-10 regulation (Figure 2). The lack of NFIL3 leads to spontaneous colitis while proper functioning of lymphocytes protects from the disease (Kobayashi et al., 2014).

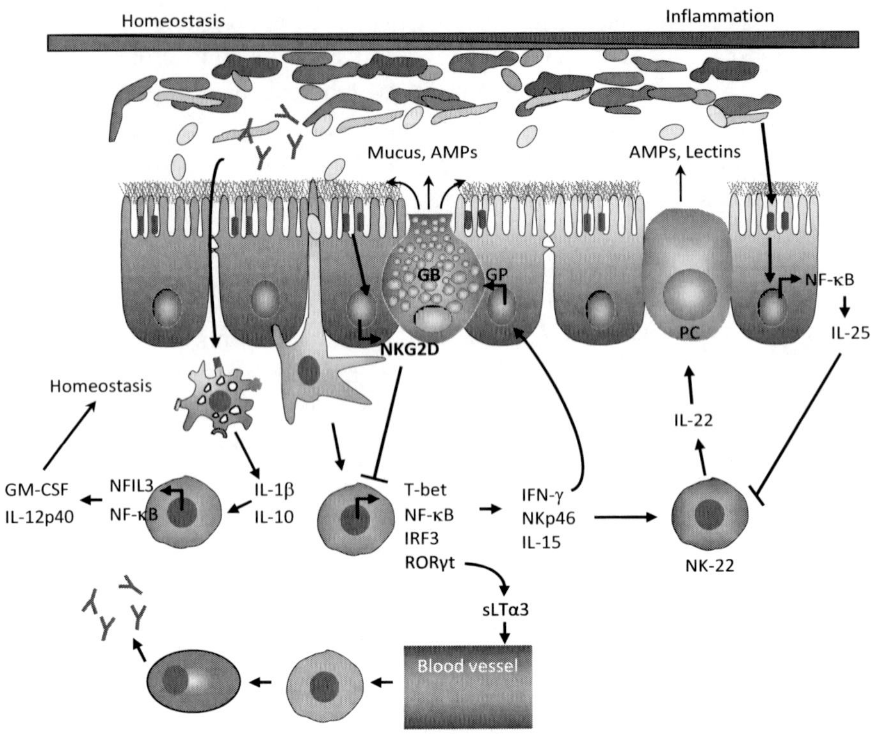

Figure 2. Influence of microbiota to innate lymphoid cells. Sampling of microbiotal antigens by dendritic cells or macrophages induces activation of various transcription factors whose effector products generate homeostatic and inflammatory responses to maintain intestinal immunity. Responses for homeostasis include production of GM-CSF, immunoglobulins following intestinal homing of B and plasma cells, mucus, and AMPs. To curb inflammation, the microbiota suppresses the inflammatory responses by suppressing the activities of ILCs such as production of IL-22, AMPs and lectins. AMPs, antimicrobial peptides; GB, goblet cell; GM-CSF, granulocyte-macrophage colony-stimulating factor; GP, glycoproteins; IRF, interferon-regulatory factors; IL, interleukin; NF-κB, nuclear factor kappa B; NK, natural killer; NKG2D, natural killer group 2 member D; PC, Paneth cell; ROR, retinoic acid orphan receptor; sLT, soluble lymphotoxin.

The ILCs also control microbiota composition through modulation of IgA production. This occurs when RORγt$^+$ ILCs produce either soluble lymphotoxin α (sLTα3) which controls T cell-dependent IgA induction via regulation of T cell homing to the gut or membrane-bound lymphotoxin β (LTα1β2) which drives T cell-independent IgA induction by controlling DC functions (Figure 2). Ablation of LTα in RORγt$^+$ cells abrogates IgA production and alters intestinal microbiota composition (Kruglov et al., 2013). It is interesting to note that the intestinal microbiota stabilizes the expression of RORγt in ILCs (Vonarbourg et al., 2010). In addition, both LTi cells and IL-22-producing NKp46$^+$ cells of the ILCs constitutively produce most of the intestinal IL-22. The microbiota represses this production by inducing epithelial expression of IL-25. This function plays an essential role in fine tuning the equilibrium among intestinal symbionts, adaptive immunity and RORγt$^+$ ILCs (Sawa et al., 2011). Maintaining microbial composition, both qualitatively and quantitatively is pivotal to gut immune homeostasis.

The microbiota also maintains production of NK for sustained gut immunity. This is exemplifies by some specific microbiota strains like *Bifidobacterium longum* BB536 which have been shown to maintain or increase the activity of NK cells in elderly which under normal circumstances decreases with aging (Akatsu et al., 2013). Increased growth of intestinal *Bifidobacterium* spp by galacto-oligosaccharides (GOS) also increases the percentage of NK cells in mesenteric lymph nodes (MLNs) and reduces severity of *Helicobacter hepaticus* colitis. In addition, GOS stimulates intestinal IL-15 production and NK expression of CCR9 designated for lymphocyte trafficking to infected areas (Gopalakrishnan et al., 2012). The increase in NK cells has also been demonstrated in a randomized, double-blinded, placebo-controlled human clinical trial carried out in 40 healthy adults. The study reported that *Lactobacillus salivarius* CECT5713 isolated from breast milk and taken orally at 2 x 10^8 colon forming units (cfu) daily for 4 weeks increases the percentage of NK cells and the regulatory cytokine IL-10 (Sierra et al., 2010). The microbiota-mediated increase in NK cells could benefit patients from several disease conditions, such as IBD in which NK cells play a role.

Microbiota-Driven ILC Functions during Disease

The potential of microbiota-NK interaction in overcoming diseases is manifested in various ways. A recent study by Klose and others (2013) reported that during ontogeny CCR6$^+$RORγt$^+$ ILCs do not express transcription factor T-bet. Instead, T-bet expression occurs in postnatal period and is controlled by signals from microbiota and IL-23. Its expression activates T-bet target genes including IFN-γ and natural cytotoxicity receptor NKp46 to produce NK-22 cells (i.e., IL-22 producing NK cells). The produced IFN-γ protects the gut against *Salmonella* enteric infection through the release of mucus-forming glycoproteins (Figure 2). The microbiota also promotes production of type I IFN by macrophages and the subsequent IFN-priming of NK cells. The primed NK cells confer protection against mouse cytomegalovirus and lymphocytic choriomeningitis virus (Ganal et al., 2012).

Furthermore, the microbiota confers benefits against NK cell leukemia, a condition characterized by an expansion of these cells. The condition develops from an immune response signaling through platelet-derived growth factor (PDGF) and IL-15 to constitutively activate the NK cell expansion while dysregulating apoptosis and favoring their survival. A dysregulated sphingolipid metabolism with increased glucosylceramide synthase (GCS) expression is the cause for the disease. Maneuvers that induce NK cell apoptosis such as suppression or inhibition of GSC expression have been earmarked as potential therapeutics against the disease (Liu et al., 2010; Watters et al., 2013). A recent study by Wieland Brown and others (2013) demonstrated ability of *Bacteroides* to produce sphingolipids (ceramide phosphorylethanolamine, dihydroceramide base and glycosphingolipid α-galactosylceramide) that play role in regulating the immune system by affecting apoptosis. Such a finding suggests that microbiota could benefit against NK leukemia by inducing apoptosis.

Mast Cells

Tissue resident mast cells are derived from myeloid stem cells that form part of the immune system. They have granules containing histamine and heparin. Traditionally, mast cells are best known to mediate allergic and anaphylactic reaction. However, it is established that they also play an important role in gut innate immunity against invading pathogens (Prussin and Metcalfe 2003). It is not so long since mast cells were considered sentinels in gut immunity through their involvement in maintaining tolerance to gut microbiota and eliminating pathogens. Mast cells are located underneath the gastrointestinal epithelium, giving them a brilliant strategic location to meet their functions.

Contribution of Microbiota to Mast Cell Functioning

During early life, the microbiota sends appropriate signals that are critical for intestinal mast cell immunoregulation to protect from IgE-induced anaphylaxis. This has been observed in germ-free mice and those with low-diversity microbiota. Such animals develop high serum levels of IgE in early life due to B cell isotype switching to IgE at mucosal sites in a CD4 T-cell- and IL-4-dependent manner. The elevated IgE levels lead to increased mast-cell-surface-bound IgE and exaggerated oral-induced systemic anaphylaxis (Figure 3). This anaphylaxis can be prevented by maintaining a critical level of microbial diversity that inhibits IgE induction (Cahenzli et al., 2013).

The microbiota influences the number and activity of mast cells with impact to intestinal health. A great increase in number of mast cells in the jejunum, allergic diarrhea and elevated ovalbumin (OVA)-specific IgG1 and total IgE in blood occur in mice sensitized with OVA. These changes are coupled with disruption of gut microbiota involving a decrease in *Lactobacillus* spp in the colon (Figure 3) (Wang et al., 2013). A separate study indicated that treatment of humanized mouse model with *Lactobacillus rhamnosus* GG (GG) and *Propionibacterium freudenreichii* spp. *shermanii* JS (PJS) lowers the numbers of intestinal mast cells and down-regulates intestinal pro-inflammatory changes induced by a high-fat diet (Oksaharju et al., 2013).

The potency of microbiota in lowering the number and activity of mast cells has also been shown in antibiotic-induced alterations of microbiota in rats. These rats exhibit an increased mast cell protease II levels and higher mast cell numbers in their intestines (Nutten et al., 2007). The alterations appear to involve almost-complete eradication of *Lactobacillus* in the whole intestine and in a drastic reduction of colonic total aerobic and anaerobic bacteria, in particular *Enterobacteriacae* and *Enterococcus* (Figure 3). Recovery of these microbes could lower the number of mast cells and their activity (Schumann et al., 2005). Furthermore, during active inflammation of trinitrobenzene sulfonic acid (TNBS)-induced colitis in mice, *Lactobacillus plantarum* NCIMB8826 or probiotic mixture VSL#3c shifts the expression of colonic gene clusters related to mast cells and antimicrobial peptides towards healthy controls' profiles (Mariman et al., 2012). Indeed, from these facts, the microbiota can be employed in treating intestinal diseases associated with increased mast cell number and activity.

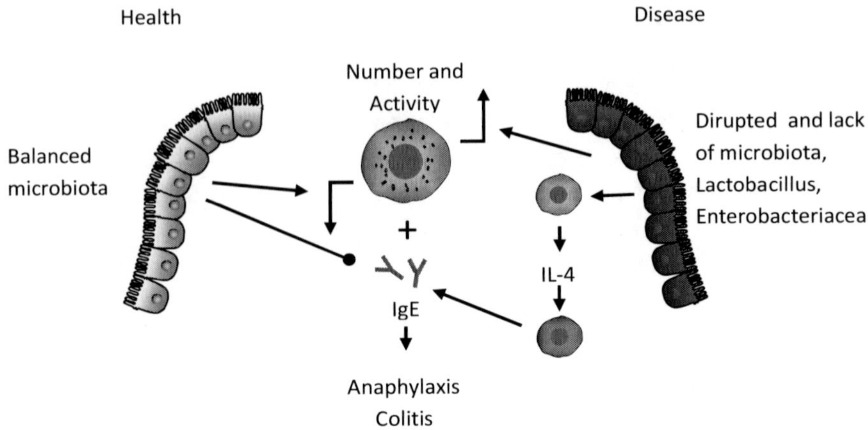

Figure 3. Influence of microbiota to mast cell functioning during health and disease. A balanced intestinal microbiota lowers the number and activity of mast cell and IgE. This reduces the mast cell binding to IgE and prevents diseases like anaphylaxis and colitis. Microbiotal disruption or absence increases mast cell number and activity as well as IgE and leads to diseases. IgE, immunoglobulin E; IL, interleukin.

Microbiota-Driven Mast Cell Function during Disease

Microbiota dysbiosis, such as small intestinal bacterial overgrowth (SIBO) and changes in the composition of the luminal and mucosal colonic microbiota have been linked to IBS. Subsets of patients with IBS show high numbers of mucosal mast cells in the small and large intestine. The mast cells have increased release of proteases, histamine, and prostanoids that contribute to perpetuation of the disease (Ortiz-Lucas et al., 2010; Barbara et al., 2011; Barbara et al., 2012). The increase in mast cells could partly be due to both psychological and physical stress. Stress induces degranulation of mucosal mast cells whose released products increase intestinal epithelial permeability. The increased permeability allows bacteria and/or their products like peptidoglycan to translocate from the lumen to the interior of the body where they prime the innate immune system to respond to antigenic stimulation. Treatments modulating the microbiota and those targeting activated mast cells may benefit IBS patients. In fact, several probiotics have shown a reduction in IBS symptoms by an immunomodulatory and analgesic effects while others have demonstrated possible benefit of microbiota-mast cell interaction to IBS. The benefits of microbiota could be related to its influence on mast cell degranulation since exposure of mast cells to microbiota down-regulates degranulation. This effect requires a direct contact between bacteria and mast cells (Wesolowski and Paumet 2011). The microbiota can also strengthern epithelial tight junctions to prevent the disease (Figure 4) (Malago 2014). Despite accumulating data on the therapeutic potential of microbiota to IBS, the pathology of the disease is complex and the available microbiotal therapeutic evidence is still weak. Thus larger trials are needed to elucidate the exact microbiota based therapeutic regime (Dahlqvist and Piessevaux 2011; Spiller and Lam 2011).

The involvement of microbial-mast cell interaction in Crohn's disease has scantly been reported. In this regard, the microbiota LPS (under dysbiosis) activates mast cells to produce IL-1β and chemokine CXCL8. This is via soluble CD14 distributed by other LPS-triggered cells at the gastrointestinal barrier. In the absence of CD14, LPS fails to stimulate mast cell expression of these mediators in both normal and Crohn's disease tissues (Brenner et al., 2014). More research is needed to elucidate further the involvement of microbiotal-mast cell interaction to Crohn's disease and other forms of IBD caused by dysbiosis of the microbiota.

EOSINOPHILS

Eosinophils are granulocytes derived during hematopoiesis in bone marrow. They differentiate from myeloid precursor cells in response to type 2 cytokines (IL-3, IL-5, and GM-CSF) (Metcalf et al., 1986, 1987; Yamaguchi et al., 1988). After maturation, they circulate in blood and migrate to inflammatory or helminth infected sites in response to chemokines (e.g., CCL5, CCL11, and CCL24) and leukotriens (LT) (e.g., LTB4) and MCP1/4 (Bandeira-Melo et al., 2002). In these sites, eosinophils are activated to produce various effector products including cationic granule proteins, RNases, reactive oxygen species (such as hypobromite, superoxide, peroxide), lipid mediators like eicosanoids from leukotriens and prostaglandins, enzymes like elastase, growth factors like transforming growth factor (TGF)-β, vascular endothelial growth factor (VEGF) and PDGF and cytokines (e.g., IL-1, IL-2, IL-4, IL-5, IL-6, IL-8, IL-13, TNF-α (Horiuchi and Weller 1997; Bandeira-Melo et al., 2002; Saito et al., 2004; Kato et al., 2005; Lacy 2005; Rothenberg and Hogan 2006; Trulson et al., 2007; Hogan et al., 2008).

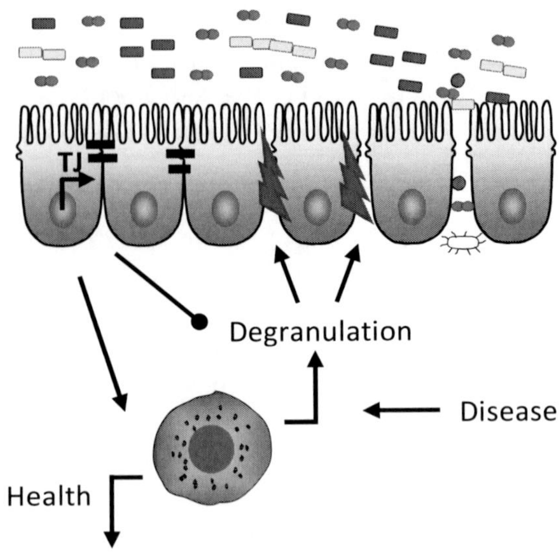

Figure 4. Microbiotal influence on mast cell-induced tight junction disruption. Increased number and degranulation of mast cells disrupts epithelial tight junctions leading to translocation of enteral antigens into submucosa to cause diseases like irritable bowel syndrome. Improvement of microbiota profile to such patients reduces the number of mast cells and degranulation, strengthens the tight junctions and benefits patients against such diseases.

Classically, eosinophils are responsible for combating multicellular parasites such as helminthes and certain infections as well as controlling allergic reactions. However, it is evident that they are involved in other biological processes including neoplasia and antigen presentation to T cells. Large numbers of eosinophils are present in the intestinal lamina propria under normal conditions with little knowledge on their exact role in mucosal immunity at steady state.

Microbiota Influence on Eosinophils

The microbiota drives some eosinophil functions including maintanace of gut homeostasis, prevention of allergic reactions and neoplasia. For maintenance of gut immune homeostasis, the microbiota drives DCs to present tolerogenic signals by expressing TNF receptor (TNFR)-associated factor (TRAF)6 molecule. DC expression of TRAF6 is pivotal to gut-microbiota dependent immune tolerance which, in part, involves inactive eosinophils.

Deletion of TRAF6 results in loss of mucosal tolerance exhibited by development of Th2 cells in the lamina propria and eosinophilic enteritis and fibrosis in the small intestine. This loss of tolerance is microbiota-dependent but independent of DC-expressed myeloid differentiation factor (MyD)88 (Han et al., 2013). The microbiota is further known to promote T-independent IgA class switching through their secreted products. Mice deficient in eosinophils exhibit impaired intestinal IgA production, accompanied by a disrupted mucosal layer and alterations in microbiota density and composition (Chu et al., 2014). The role played by eosinophils in maintaining immune homeostasis in the gut revolves around influencing functional crosstalk between microbiota, IgA, T cells, and DCs (Figure 5). Studies involving eosinophil-deficient and eosinophil-specific depletion mice models have shown reduced IgA plasma cell numbers and secreted IgA, defects in intestinal mucous shield, alterations in microbiota composition, and disturbed TGF-β-dependent class switching to IgA in Peyer's patches, formation of $CD103^+$ T cells like $Foxp3^+$ regulatory cells, and $CD103^+$ DCs in these mice (Chu et al., 2014). Together, these results clearly indicate the microbiota-eosinophil interaction to maintain the gut immune homeostasis via modulation of the key immune system components.

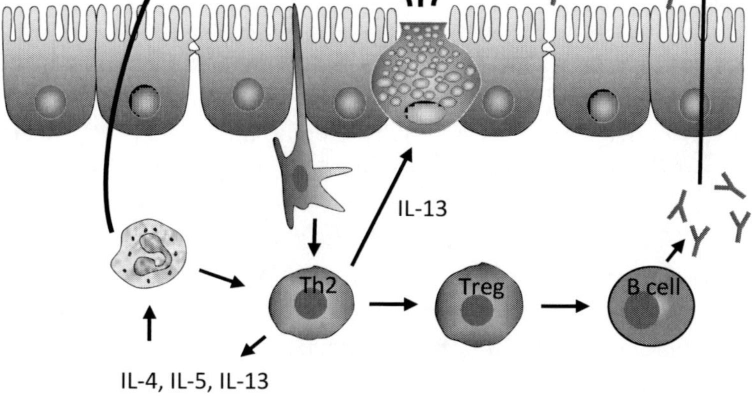

Figure 5. Microbiota-eosinophil interaction for intestinal immunity. Microbiota, sampled by dendritic cells influence eosinophil production and functions. Part of eosinophils' functions includes regulation of luminal microbiota profile directly or through production of immunoglobulins. IL, interleukin; Th, T helper; Treg, T regulatory.

Microbiota-Driven Eosinophil Functions during Disease

There is enough evidence on the influence of microbiota to eosinophils on controlling allergic reactions. A study by Bisgaard and others (2011) showed that microbiotal diversity of neonates at 1 and 12 months of age is inversely associated with the risk of allergic sensitization, peripheral blood eosinophils, and allergic rhinitis in the first 6 years of life. The increase in eosinophilia due to poor microbial diversity could result in serious inflammatory reactions in various tissues. Specific microbes have been implicated in affecting eosinophil production and functions to alleviate allergic reactions in animal models and humans. For example oral administration of microbiotal bacterial strains *Bifidobacterium breve* M-16V and *Lactobacillus plantarum* NumRes8 to OVA-sensitized BALB/c mice reduces the number of eosinophils in the bronchoalveolar lavage fluid as well as OVA-specific IgE and IgG1 and prevents development of allergic reactions in these animals (Hougee et al., 2010). Similarly, combined administration of *Lactobacillus acidophilus* NCFM and *Bifidobacterium lactis* Bl-04 prevents pollen-induced infiltration of eosinophils into the nasal mucosa of children. In these children, pollen season induces a reduction in *Bifidobacterium, Clostridium* and *Bacteroides*. Although the reduced commensals are not recovered by this treatment, the administered microbiota member species are able to prevent the allergic reactions by suppressing eosinophil production and function (Ouwehand et al., 2009).

Although literature is scarce on the effect of microbiota-eosinophil interaction on neoplasia, there is a possibility that this interaction benefits cancer patients. Eosinophils have been shown to play role in development of colon polyposis and cancer. A study by Dennis and others (2013) indicated that disrupted microbiota characterized by high densities of microbes, results in development of colon polyposis with densely eosinophilic infiltrated polyps. The nature of eosinophil infiltration was in a similar way to that caused by enrichment of polyps by microbiota associated previously with colon cancer. These observations could mean that disruption of intestinal microbiota triggers production of eosinophils that may drive colon polyps and/or cancer development. Maintaining proper microbial balance could benefit against these disorders.

BASOPHILS

Basophils are granulocytic leukocytes often found in circulation. They are the least common of the circulating leukocytes. They are similar to mast cells in function though they arise from different cell lines. Contrary to mast cells, basophils remain in circulation unless needed to be recruited into tissue out of the blood flow. Basophil granules contain pre-stored proteoglycans (i.e., chondroitin and anticoagulant heparin) and histamine which dilates blood vessels and promotes blood flow to tissues. They also secrete newly synthesized substances including proteolytic enzymes such as elastase and lysophospholipase and mediators like leukotrienes and cytokines (Smith et al., 2012).

Basophils execute pro-inflammatory effector function during allergy and ectoparasite infection. They contain receptors for IgE, produce IL-4, and regulate Th2 responses that mediate parasitic defense and allergic reactions (Smith et al., 2012; Noti et al., 2014). Furthermore, there is enough evidence that basophils are antigen presenting cells capable of inducing Th2 cells both in vitro and in vivo. They express MHCII and CD80/86 required for antigen presentation. Thus they can take-up antigens, especially antigen (Ag)-IgE complexes, process them, and present peptide with MHCII to Th cells (Nakanishi 2010).

Microbiota-Basophil Interaction

The microbiota-basophil interaction for gut immunity has not been established. There is scant information on the influence of microbiota to basophil functioning in other body systems which could be suggestive of a more or less similar benefit to the gut. For instance, microbiota has been shown to influence immune response involving basophils in chronic rhinosinusitis (CRS). This was demonstrated in a case versus control study involving 30 patients with CRS and 12 healthy controls undergoing surgery. The study assessed immune response of peripheral blood leukocytes to lavage microbiota. It was established that CRS patients have a quantitative but not qualitative increase in the number of microbiota species, increase in the levels of eosinophils and basophils as well as the corresponding cytokines IL-4, IL-5, IL-8, and IL-13 in their lavage. The increased basophils could be due to immune hyperresponsiveness to commensal organisms (Aurora et al., 2013). Suppressing basophil responses or depletion of basophils has been shown to reduce susceptibility to intestinal food allergy (Noti et al., 2014). There is a need for more research to explore the microbiota-basophil interaction for gut immunity to establish the beneficial microbial profile that will form basis for designing therapeutics against microbiota-eosinophil mediated diseases.

PHAGOCYTIC CELLS: NEUTROPHILS

Neutrophils are the most abundant white blood cells in human and most animals. They are normally found in blood vessels from which they migrate to areas of insult to phagocytose bacteria and cause inflammation. Their phagocytic capacity to engulf bacteria is affected by simple sugars, of which they have a preference to engulf over bacteria, but strengthened by fasting (Sanchez et al., 1973). Interestingly, this phagocytic capacity is augmented after translocation of neutrophils into the intestinal lumen where they exhibit a dramatic increase in the level of CD11b/CD18, elevated preservation of superoxide production and increased killing of microbes like *Salmonella typhimurium* (Hofman et al., 2000; Nadeau et al., 2002). Neutrophils are highly motile. They quickly congregate at a focus of infection following attraction by chemotactic cytokines like IL-8 and TNF-α that direct the path of their migration. They can also express and produce cytokines that recruit and activate other immune cells to amplify inflammatory reactions. The killing of bacteria by neutrophils is in three categories: they can directly attack micro-organisms by phagocytosis, they can release antimicrobials and proteolytic enzymes from their granules, and can generate neutrophil extracellular traps (NETs).

Phagocytosis of antigens follows opsonization of microbes and other potentially harmful particles. A phagosome is formed to contain the engulfed material prior to fusing with a lysosome. The latter pours its reactive oxygen species (respiratory burst) and hydrolytic enzymes to kill the microbes. During respiratory burst, NADPH oxidase is activated to release superoxide that either decays spontaneously or is broken down by superoxide dismutases to hydrogen peroxide. The generated hydrogen peroxide reacts with myeloperoxidase to produce hypochlorous acid whose bactericidal activity kills the engulfed microbes (Segal 2005). Various antimicrobials and proteolytic enzymes are released by neutrophils during degranulation to destroy microbes or institute intended immune function. They include myeloperoxidase, bactericidal/permeability-increasing protein (BPI), defensins, cathepsin, gelatinase, cathelicidin, collagenase, alkaline phosphatase, lysozyme, NADPH oxidase, serine proteases, and neutrophil elastase. The role of these antimicrobial proteins and enzymes is to combat microbes and restore gut innate immunity.

NETs are web-like structures made of chromatin and serine proteases. They are produced following activation of neutrophils to trap and kill microbes extracellularly, particularly large-sized pathogens like *Candida albicans* hyphae and extracellular aggregates of *Mycobacterium bovis* (Branzk et al., 2014). Literature is still scant on how NETs carry out their functions. Nonetheless, they may provide a high local concentration of antimicrobials that kill microbes independent of phagocytosis. They also serve as a physical barrier to prevent spread of pathogens (Branzk et al., 2014; Manfredi et al., 2014).

Microbiota and Neutrophils for Gut Immunity during Health and Disease

Entry of pathogens to the gut, challenges the immune system, including the microbiota and neutrophils, in an attempt to establish in the host. Sometimes the pathogen succeeds in breaking the immunity by negatively impacting the immune system. For instance, *Salmonella enterica* serovar Typhimurium infection in mice causes recruitment of neutrophils to the gut lumen. The recruited neutrophils produce elastase that induces significant changes in intestinal microbiota composition, including reduction in the total number of microbiota and depletion or reduction of *Ruminococcaceae* and *Lachnospiraceae* family members. The elastase-induced microbiotal changes favor *Salmonella* colonization (Sekirov et al., 2010; Gill et al., 2012). Further, intestinal *Salmonella* infection induces respiratory burst of neutrophils that oxidizes endogenous sulfur compounds to generate a respiratory electron acceptor, tetrathionate (Figure 6). The generated tetrathionate respiration is used by *Salmonella* to outgrow the microbiota in the anaerobic intestinal environment leading to expedited transmission of the pathogen (Winter and Bäumler 2011).

Despite some failures in the immune system to curb pathogenic invasion, there is enough evidence indicating the beneficial role of microbiota-driven neutrophil function against pathogens. This has been demonstrated under various conditions. For instance animals without endogenous intestinal microbiota are highly susceptible to primary intracellular infection by pathogenic *Listeria monocytogenes* with impaired activation and accumulation of phagocytes to the site of infection (Mittrücker et al., 2014). Clarke and others (2010) observed that microbiota peptidoglycan signaling through Nod1 systemically primes the innate immune system to enhance killing of pathogenic *Streptococcus pneumoniae* and *Staphylococcus aureus* by neutrophils (Figure 6) (Clarke et al., 2010). Another study indicated that the microbiota shapes the neutrophil oxidative reactions to kill pathogens. This is exemplified by *L. rhamnosus* GG which potently dampens production of reactive oxygen species and phagocytic capacity of the neutrophils while protecting against cell cytotoxicity. By so doing, the microbiota confers desensitization towards luminal antigens, favors survival of beneficial microbes that contribute to maintenance of gut immunity (Vong et al., 2014).

Sometimes encounter of pathogens by neutrophils induces formation of NETs that are used to effectively capture, contain, and kill microorganisms. The function of NETs is well regulated since excessive or uncontrolled production of NETs damages surrounding cells and predisposes to gastrointestinal diseases. Interestingly, the microbiota, at least in part, contributes to this regulation. This has recently been shown by Vong and others (2014) who observed that *Lactobacillus rhamnosus* GG inhibits both phorbol 12-myristate 13-acetate- and *Staphylococcus aureus*-induced formation of NETs. This inhibitory regulation could favor appropriate destruction of the pathogen by neutrophils.

The beneficial role of microbiota-neutrophil interaction has also been observed under conditions of antibiotic-induced dysbiosis. Prolonged duration of antibiotic therapy that disrupts the microbiota predisposes neonates to late-onset sepsis (LOS), a disorder controlled by neutrophils. The microbiota plays essential role in regulating neutrophils to curb LOS. The regulation is depicted by induction of IL-17 production by intestinal ILCs, increased plasma granulocyte colony-stimulating factor (G-CSF) levels and neutrophil numbers in a toll-like receptor 4- and MyD88-dependent manner and restoration of IL-17-dependent resistance to LOS. Deletion of ILCs prevents IL-17- and G-CSF-dependent granulocytosis and resistance to LOS (Deshmukh et al., 2014).

Phagocytic Cells: Macrophages and DCs

The mononuclear phagocytes macrophages and DCs, are pivotal to the trafficking of innate immune signals to the adaptive immunity to mount responses. They do not fully qualify as components of the innate immune system. Instead, they are at the interface between innate and adaptive immune systems. For this reason, they will be discussed in a separate chapter.

CONCLUSION

Microbiotal shaping of cells of the innate immune system is a great potential to developing medicaments that will treat intestinal disorders caused by disrupted commensals. Although at the moment there is no substantial therapeutic regime based on microbiotal-mediated shaping of innate immune cells, the microbiota-innate immune cell interaction described in this chapter indicates clearly that such an approach is possible. The approach can focus on strengthening the influence of microbiota on innate immune cells. This could subsequently improve intestinal immunity during health and control inflammatory reactions during disease without much tissue damage.

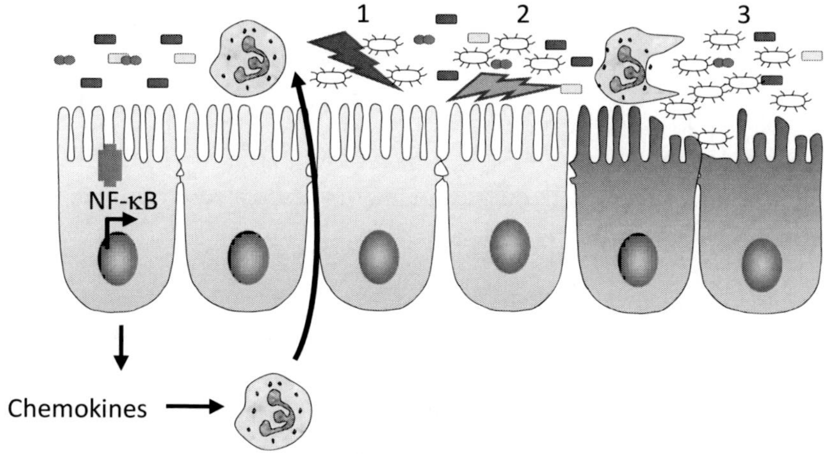

Figure 6. Microbiotal influence on neutrophil functioning for intestinal immunity. A balanced microbiota activates transcription factors to produce chemokines that attract neutrophils to infected sites. Attracted neutrophils destroy pathogens (1) such as *Streptococcus species* and *Staphylococcus aureus*. The microbiota also prevents infection (2) by some intestinal pathogens such as *Listeria monocytogenes*. Pathogens like *Salmonella* may disrupt microbiota profile and utilize neutrophil respiratory burst to cause disease (3).

REFERENCES

Akatsu, H; Iwabuchi, N; Xiao, JZ; et al. Clinical effects of probiotic Bifidobacterium longum BB536 on immune function and intestinal microbiota in elderly patients receiving enteral tube feeding. *JPEN J Parenter Enteral Nutr.*, 2013, 37, 631-640.

Aurora, R; Chatterjee, D; Hentzleman, J; et al. Contrasting the microbiomes from healthy volunteers and patients with chronic rhinosinusitis. *JAMA Otolaryngol Head Neck Surg.*, 2013, 139, 1328-1338.

Bandeira-Melo, C; Bozza, PT; Weller, PF. The cellular biology of eosinophil eicosanoid formation and function. *J Allergy Clin Immunol.*, 2002, 109, 393-400.

Barbara, G; Cremon, C; Carini, G; et al. The immune system in irritable bowel syndrome. *J Neurogastroenterol Motil.*, 2011, 17, 349-359.

Barbara, G; Zecchi, L; Barbaro, R; et al. Mucosal permeability and immune activation as potential therapeutic targets of probiotics in irritable bowel syndrome. *J Clin Gastroenterol.*, 2012, 46 Suppl, S52-5.

Bhatnagar, N; Ahmad, F; Hong, HS; et al. FcγRIII (CD16)-mediated ADCC by NK cells is regulated by monocytes and FcγRII (CD32). *Eur J Immunol.*, 2014, In press.

Bisgaard, H; Li, N; Bonnelykke, K; Chawes, BL; et al. Reduced diversity of the intestinal microbiota during infancy is associated with increased risk of allergic disease at school age. *J Allergy Clin Immunol.*, 2011, 128, 646-652.

Branzk, N; Lubojemska, A; Hardison, SE; et al. Neutrophils sense microbe size and selectively release neutrophil extracellular traps in response to large pathogens. *Nat Immunol.*, 2014, In press.

Brenner, SA; Zacheja, S; Schäffer, M; et al. Soluble CD14 is essential for lipopolysaccharide-dependent activation of human intestinal mast cells from macroscopically normal as well as Crohn's disease tissue. *Immunology.*, 2014, 143, 174-183.

Cahenzli, J; Köller, Y; Wyss, M; et al. Intestinal microbial diversity during early-life colonization shapes long-term IgE levels. *Cell Host Microbe.*, 2013, 14, 559-570.

Campos, C; Pera, A; Sanchez-Correa, B; et al. Effect of age and CMV on NK cell subpopulations. *Exp Gerontol.*, 2014, 54, 130-137.

Chu, VT; Beller, A; Rausch, S; et al. Eosinophils promote generation and maintenance of immunoglobulin-A-expressing plasma cells and contribute to gut immune homeostasis. *Immunity.*, 2014, 40, 582-593.

Clarke, TB; Davis, KM; Lysenko, ES; et al. Recognition of peptidoglycan from the microbiota by Nod1 enhances systemic innate immunity. *Nat Med.*, 2010, 16, 228-231.

Dahlqvist, G; Piessevaux, H. Irritable bowel syndrome: the role of the intestinal microbiota, pathogenesis and therapeutic targets. *Acta Gastroenterol Belg.*, 2011, 74, 375-380.

Dennis, KL; Wang, Y; Blatner, NR; et al. Adenomatous polyps are driven by microbe-instigated focal inflammation and are controlled by IL-10-producing T cells. *Cancer Res.*, 2013, 73, 5905-5913.

Deshmukh, HS; Liu, Y; Menkiti, OR; et al. The microbiota regulates neutrophil homeostasis and host resistance to Escherichia coli K1 sepsis in neonatal mice. *Nat Med.*, 2014, 20, 524-530.

Ganal, SC; Sanos, SL; Kallfass, C; et al. Priming of natural killer cells by nonmucosal mononuclear phagocytes requires instructive signals from commensal microbiota. *Immunity.*, 2012, 37, 171-186.

Gill, N; Ferreira, RB; Antunes, LC; et al. Neutrophil elastase alters the murine gut microbiota resulting in enhanced Salmonella colonization. *PLoS One.*, 2012, 7, e49646.

Gopalakrishnan, A; Clinthorne, JF; Rondini, EA; et al. Supplementation with galacto-oligosaccharides increases the percentage of NK cells and reduces colitis severity in Smad3-deficient mice. *J Nutr.*, 2012, 142, 1336-1342.

Han, D; Walsh, MC; Cejas, PJ; et al. Dendritic cell expression of the signaling molecule TRAF6 is critical for gut microbiota-dependent immune tolerance. *Immunity.*, 2013, 27, 38, 1211-1222.

Hansen, CH; Holm, TL; Krych, Ł; et al. Gut microbiota regulates NKG2D ligand expression on intestinal epithelial cells. *Eur J Immunol.*, 2013, 43, 447-457.

Heidenreich, S; Zu, Eulenburg, C; Hildebrandt, Y; et al. Impact of the NK cell receptor LIR-1 (ILT-2/CD85j/LILRB1) on cytotoxicity against multiple myeloma. *Clin Dev Immunol.*, 2012, 2012, 652130.

Hofman, P; Piche, M; Far, DF; et al. Increased Escherichia coli phagocytosis in neutrophils that have transmigrated across a cultured intestinal epithelium. *Infect Immun.*, 2000, 68, 449-455.

Hogan, SP; Rosenberg, HF; Moqbel, R; et al. Eosinophils: biological properties and role in health and disease. *Clin Exp Allergy.*, 2008, 38, 709-750.

Horiuchi, T; Weller, PF. Expression of vascular endothelial growth factor by human eosinophils: upregulation by granulocyte macrophage colony-stimulating factor and interleukin-5. *Am J Respir Cell Mol Biol.*, 1997, 17, 70-77.

Hougee, S; Vriesema, AJ; Wijering, SC; et al. Oral treatment with probiotics reduces allergic symptoms in ovalbumin-sensitized mice: a bacterial strain comparative study. *Int Arch Allergy Immunol.*, 2010, 151, 107-117.

Kato, Y; Fujisawa, T; Nishimori, H; et al. Leukotriene D4 induces production of transforming growth factor-beta1 by eosinophils. *Int Arch Allergy Immunol.*, 2005, 137 Suppl 1, 17-20.

Klose, CS; Kiss, EA; Schwierzeck, V; et al. A T-bet gradient controls the fate and function of CCR6-RORγt+ innate lymphoid cells. *Nature.*, 2013, 494, 261-265.

Knoop, KA; McDonald, KG; McCrate, S; et al. Microbial sensing by goblet cells controls immune surveillance of luminal antigens in the colon. *Mucosal Immunol.*, 2014, In press.

Kobayashi, T; Steinbach, EC; Russo, SM; et al. NFIL3-deficient mice develop microbiota-dependent, IL-12/23-driven spontaneous colitis. *J Immunol.*, 2014, 192, 1918-1927.

Kruglov, AA; Grivennikov, SI; Kuprash, DV; et al. Nonredundant function of soluble LTα3 produced by innate lymphoid cells in intestinal homeostasis. *Science.*, 2013, 342, 1243-1246.

Kruse, PH; Matta, J; Ugolini, S; et al. Natural cytotoxicity receptors and their ligands. *Immunol Cell Biol.*, 2014 Mar, 92(3), 221-9

Lacy, P. The role of Rho GTPases and SNAREs in mediator release from granulocytes. *Pharmacol Ther.*, 2005, 107, 358-376.

Liu, X; Ryland, L; Yang, J; et al. Targeting of survivin by nanoliposomal ceramide induces complete remission in a rat model of NK-LGL leukemia. *Blood.*, 2010, 116, 4192-4201.

Malago, JJ. Contribution of microbiota to the intestinal physicochemical barrier. *Benef Microbes.*, 2014, In press.

Manfredi, AA; Covino, C; Rovere-Querini, P; et al. Instructive influences of phagocytic clearance of dying cells on neutrophil extracellular trap generation. *Clin Exp Immunol.*, 2014, In press.

Mariman, R; Kremer, B; van, Erk, M; et al. Gene expression profiling identifies mechanisms of protection to recurrent trinitrobenzene sulfonic acid colitis mediated by probiotics. *Inflamm Bowel Dis.*, 2012, 18, 1424-1433.

Metcalf, D; Begley, CG; Nicola, NA; et al. Quantitative responsiveness of murine hemopoietic populations in vitro and in vivo to recombinant multi-CSF (IL-3). *Exp Hematol.*, 1987, 15, 288-295.

Metcalf, D; Burgess, AW; Johnson, GR; et al. In vitro actions on hemopoietic cells of recombinant murine GM-CSF purified after production in Escherichia coli: comparison with purified native GM-CSF. *J Cell Physiol.*, 1986, 128, 421-431.

Mittrücker, HW; Seidel, D; Bland, PW; et al. Lack of microbiota reduces innate responses and enhances adaptive *immunity* against Listeria monocytogenes infection. *Eur J Immunol.*, 2014, 44, 1710-1715.

Mortha, A; Chudnovskiy, A; Hashimoto, D; et al. Microbiota-dependent crosstalk between macrophages and ILC3 promotes intestinal homeostasis. *Science.*, 2014, 343, 1249288.

Nadeau, WJ; Pistole, TG; McCormick, BA. Polymorphonuclear leukocyte migration across model intestinal epithelia enhances Salmonella typhimurium killing via the epithelial derived cytokine, IL-6. *Microbes Infect.*, 2002, 4, 1379-1387.

Nakanishi, K. Basophils as APC in Th2 response in allergic inflammation and parasite infection. *Curr Opin Immunol.*, 2010, 22, 814-820.

Neill, DR; Wong, SH; Bellosi, A; et al. Nuocytes represent a new innate effector leukocyte that mediates type-2 immunity. *Nature.*, 2010, 464, 1367-1370.

Noti, M; Kim, BS; Siracusa, MC; et al. Exposure to food allergens through inflamed skin promotes intestinal food allergy through the thymic stromal lymphopoietin-basophil axis. *J Allergy Clin Immunol.*, 2014, 133, 1390-1399.

Nutten, S; Schumann, A; Donnicola, D; et al. Antibiotic administration early in life impairs specific humoral responses to an oral antigen and increases intestinal mast cell numbers and mediator concentrations. *Clin Vaccine Immunol.*, 2007, 14, 190-197.

Oksaharju, A; Kooistra, T; Kleemann, R; et al. Effects of probiotic Lactobacillus rhamnosus GG and Propionibacterium freudenreichii ssp. shermanii JS supplementation on intestinal and systemic markers of inflammation in ApoE*3Leiden mice consuming a high-fat diet. *Br J Nutr.*, 2013, 110, 77-85.

Ortiz-Lucas, M; Saz-Peiró, P; Sebastián-Domingo, JJ. Irritable bowel syndrome immune hypothesis. Part one: the role of lymphocytes and mast cells. *Rev Esp Enferm Dig.*, 2010, 102, 637-647.

Ouwehand, AC; Nermes, M; Collado, MC; et al. Specific probiotics alleviate allergic rhinitis during the birch pollen season. *World J Gastroenterol.*, 2009, 15, 3261-3268.

Prussin, C; Metcalfe, DD. 4. IgE, mast cells, basophils, and eosinophils. *J Allergy Clin Immunol.*, 2003, 111, S486-94.

Review. Erratum in: *J Allergy Clin Immunol.*, 2003, 112, 267.

Rothenberg, ME; Hogan, SP. The eosinophil. *Annu Rev Immunol.*, 2006, 24, 147-174.

Saito, K; Nagata, M; Kikuchi, I; et al. Leukotriene D4 and eosinophil transendothelial migration, superoxide generation, and degranulation via beta2 integrin. *Ann Allergy Asthma Immunol.*, 2004, 93, 594-600.

Sanchez, A; Reeser, JL; Lau, HS; et al. Role of sugars in human neutrophilic phagocytosis. *Am J Clin Nutr.*, 1973, 26, 1180-1184.

Sawa, S; Lochner, M; Satoh-Takayama, N; et al. RORγt+ innate lymphoid cells regulate intestinal homeostasis by integrating negative signals from the symbiotic microbiota. *Nat Immunol.*, 2011, 12, 320-326.

Schumann, A; Nutten, S; Donnicola, D; et al. Neonatal antibiotic treatment alters gastrointestinal tract developmental gene expression and intestinal barrier transcriptome. *Physiol Genomics.*, 2005, 23, 235-245.

Segal, AW. How neutrophils kill microbes. *Annu Rev Immunol.*, 2005, 9, 197–223.

Sekirov, I; Gill, N; Jogova, M; et al. Salmonella SPI-1-mediated neutrophil recruitment during enteric colitis is associated with reduction and alteration in intestinal microbiota. *Gut Microbes.*, 2010, 1, 30-41.

Sierra, S; Lara-Villoslada, F; Sempere, L; et al. Intestinal and immunological effects of daily oral administration of Lactobacillus salivarius CECT5713 to healthy adults. *Anaerobe.*, 2010, 16, 195-200.

Smith, KA; Harcus, Y; Garbi, N; et al. Type 2 innate *immunity* in helminth infection is induced redundantly and acts autonomously following CD11c(+) cell depletion. *Infect Immun.*, 2012, 80, 3481-3489.

Spiller, R; Lam, C. The shifting interface between IBS and IBD. *Curr Opin Pharmacol.*, 2011, 11, 586-592.

Spits, H; Di, Santo, JP. The expanding family of innate lymphoid cells: regulators and effectors of *immunity* and tissue remodeling. *Nat Immunol.*, 2011, 12, 21-27.

Trulson, A; Byström, J; Engström, A; et al. The functional heterogeneity of eosinophil cationic protein is determined by a gene polymorphism and post-translational modifications. *Clin Exp Allergy.*, 2007, 37, 208-218.

Tu, MM; Mahmoud, AB; Wight, A; et al. Ly49 family receptors are required for cancer immunosurveillance mediated by natural killer cells. *Cancer Res.*, 2014, 74, 3684-3694.

Vivier, E; Raulet, DH; Moretta, A; et al. Innate or Adaptive *Immunity*? The Example of Natural Killer Cells. *Science*, 2011, 331, 44–49.

Vonarbourg, C; Mortha, A; Bui, VL; et al. Regulated expression of nuclear receptor RORγt confers distinct functional fates to NK cell receptor-expressing RORγt(+) innate lymphocytes. *Immunity*., 2010, 33, 736-751.

Vong, L; Lorentz, RJ; Assa, A; et al. Probiotic Lactobacillus rhamnosus inhibits the formation of neutrophil extracellular traps. *J Immunol.*, 2014, 192, 1870-1877.

Walker, JA; Barlow, JL; McKenzie, AN. Innate lymphoid cells--how did we miss them? *Nat Rev Immunol.,* 2013, 13, 75-87.

Walker, JA; Barlow, JL; McKenzie, ANJ. Innate lymphoid cells – how did we miss them? *Nature Reviews Immunology*, 2013, 13, 75-87.

Wang, JH; Fan, SW; Zhu, WY. Development of Gut Microbiota in a Mouse Model of Ovalbumin-induced Allergic Diarrhea under Sub-barrier System. *Asian-Australas J Anim Sci*., 2013, 26, 545-551.

Watters, RJ; Fox, TE; Tan, SF; et al. Targeting glucosylceramide synthase synergizes with C6-ceramide nanoliposomes to induce apoptosis in natural killer cell leukemia. *Leuk Lymphoma*., 2013, 54, 1288-1296.

Wesolowski, J; Paumet, F. The impact of bacterial infection on mast cell degranulation. *Immunol Res*., 2011, 51, 215-226.

Wieland, Brown, LC; Penaranda, C; Kashyap, PC; et al. Production of α-galactosylceramide by a prominent member of the human gut microbiota. *PLoS Biol*., 2013, 11, e1001610.

Winter, SE; Bäumler, AJ. A breathtaking feat: to compete with the gut microbiota, Salmonella drives its host to provide a respiratory electron acceptor. *Gut Microbes.*, 2011, 2, 58-60.

Withers, DR; Gaspal, FM; Mackley, EC; et al. Cutting edge: lymphoid tissue inducer cells maintain memory CD4 T cells within secondary lymphoid tissue. *J Immunol.*, 2012, 189, 2094-2098.

Yamaguchi, Y; Suda, T; Suda, J; et al. Purified interleukin 5 supports the terminal differentiation and proliferation of murine eosinophilic precursors. *J Exp Med.*, 1988, 167, 43-56.

Chapter 3

MICROBIOTAL SHAPING OF ANTIGEN PRESENTING CELL SIGNALING DURING INTESTINAL IMMUNE RESPONSE

ABSTRACT

The intestinal lumen contains diverse range of antigens from food proteins, microbiota, and pathogenic microbes that constantly challenge the immune system. While antigens from food proteins and microbiota are not harmful, those from pathogenic microbes are detrimental to the body. The immune system detects both types of antigens and drives immune responses geared at inducing tolerance or reaction to maintain immune homeostasis. Uptake of these antigens is done by professional antigen presenting cells (APCs) that include macrophages, dendritc cells (DCs) and to less extent B cells. These cells sample, phagocytose, process, and present antigens to effector cells of the adaptive immune system which generate responses corresponding to particular antigen. The microbiota influences the nature and type of responses generated by APC-activated effector cells by shaping the APC signaling to the adaptive immune system. In a steady state gut environment, the shaping is towards tolerogenic responses while a protective inflammatory reaction results from antigens sampled from harmful microbes. Thus, in an intact immune system, noxious agents like pathogens usually do not establish to cause disease. On the contrary, disruption of microbiota profile fails the shaping of appropriate protective signals from APCs leading to pro-inflammatory responses from effector cells. The end result is development of immune mediated diseases like inflammatory bowel diseases. In this chapter, recent findings on microbiota shaping of APC signaling and the resulting adaptive immune response under health and disease are discussed.

Introduction

The gastrointestinal tract is constantly exposed to an array of non-harmful antigens from food proteins and microbiota and harmful antigens from pathogenic organisms, mainly bacteria. Because of wide range of these antigens, immune responses in the gut need to be tightly regulated, especially in the colon where the pool of commensal bacteria is enormously diverse. To keep its immune homeostasis, the gut has developed mechanisms that either maintain immunological tolerance to non-harmful antigens or induce protective immune responses to eliminate pathogenic organisms (Mann et al., 2007; Amu et al., 2010; Lee et al., 2011).

The immune process starts by antigen uptake or sampling, followed by processing and presentation of the antigens to cells of the immune system before responses are induced. Antigen presentation to elicit tolerance or immune reaction in the gut is done by professional antigen presenting cells (APCs) that include macrophages, dendritic cells (DCs) and to a lesser extent B cells (Batista and Harwood 2009; Steinman 2012). These cells are pivotal to initiating, maintaining and shaping of both innate and adaptive immune systems in the gut. They link the innate and adaptive immune systems during tolerogenic or immunological reactions for gut immunity (Fujimoto et al., 2011).

The functions of APCs in intestinal innate immunity are mainly mediated through their pattern recognition receptors (PRRs) such as Toll-like receptors (TLRs) that recognize enteric antigens including microbiota antigens (Fujimoto et al., 2011). In adaptive immunity, APCs are directly involved in driving regulatory responses such as differentiation, expansion, and maintenance of regulatory T cell (Treg) populations as well as induction of immunoglobulin (Ig)A against the microbiota (Manicassamy and Pulendran, 2009). DCs in particular, drive primary T cell responses while both B cells and macrophages polarize effector T cell responses (Steinman 2012). In addition, B cells may interact directly with T cells to polarize the T cell effector responses (Batista and Harwood 2009) or produce cytokines like interleukin (IL)-10 or transforming growth factor (TGF)-β necessary for generation of Treg cells and tolerogenic responses to gut microbiota and food antigens (Figure 1) (Mann et al., 2007; Amu et al., 2010; Lee et al., 2011). Interaction of DCs or macrophages with B cells may induce differentiation of naïve B cells into immunoglobulin (Ig)A-producing plasma cells that play major role in humoral gut immunity (Fujimoto et al., 2011).

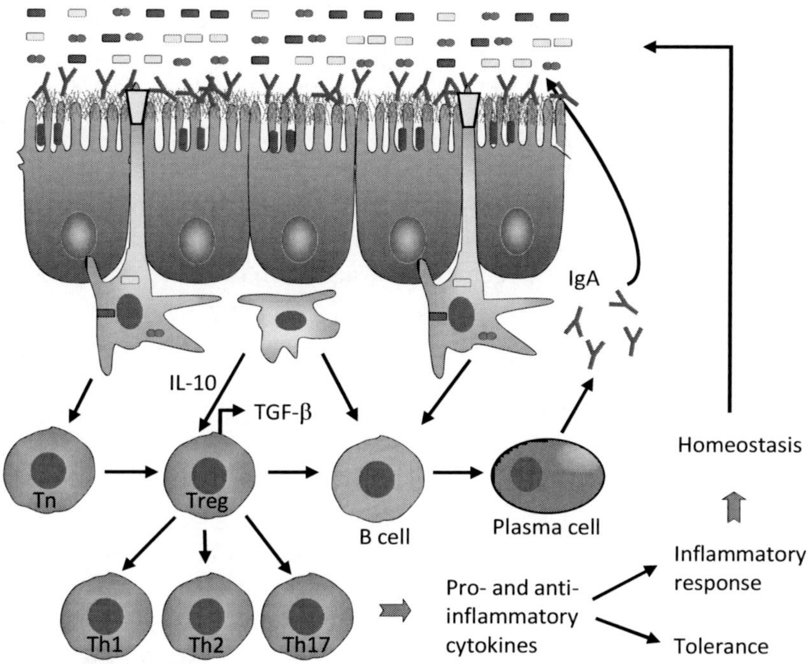

Figure 1. Microbiota-dendritic cell functioning for intestinal immunity. In a balanced microbiota, dendritic cells sample microbiotal antigens and prime naïve T cells (Tn) to differentiate into regulatory T cells (Treg), T helper (Th1, Th2, Th17) and B cells that subsequently produce immunoglobulin A (IgA). Lamina propria dendritic cells produce interleukin (IL)-10 to induce expression of transforming growth factor (TGF)-β by Treg cells to differentiate into B cells. Both effector products from Th1, Th2 and Th17 and B cell produced immunoglobulins regulate gut microbiota profile to maintain homeostasis.

The microbiota influences APC functions pertaining to intestinal immune homeostasis and responses to foster gut immunity. Imbalances of microbiota and the subsequent defective APC signaling lead to intestinal disorders such as inflammatory bowel disease (IBD) which develops due to either a mucosal susceptibility or defect in sampling of gut luminal antigens. Both events may induce TLR activity that activates innate immune response exhibited by sampling of gut antigens by APCs. Subsequently, APCs mediate the differentiation of naïve T cells into effector T helper (Th) cells, including Th1, Th2, and Th17 (Figure 1). These effectors alter the gut homeostasis and induce gastrointestinal diseases (Bermudez-Brito et al., 2014; Goto et al., 2014; Janelsins et al., 2014). In steady state gut immunity, the microbiota drives a delicate balance between pro- and anti-inflammatory mechanisms that are pivotal to immune homeostasis. This is through the ability of specific members of the microbiota to potentiate the generation of pro-inflammatory Th17 cells or anti-inflammatory Treg cells that express transcription factor Foxp3. It is the Treg cells that play a key role in limiting inflammatory responses in the intestine (Rivollier et al., 2012; Arpaia et al., 2013).

Several studies have demonstrated the potential of microbiatal shaping of APC signaling to influence effector responses (Rivollier et al., 2012; Shaw et al., 2012; Rodes et al., 2013; Trapecar et al., 2014). In general terms, an intact normal microbiota profile shapes the APC-mediated signaling towards maintenance of gut immune homeostasis. This is through inducing tolerogenic responses towards harmless antigens from food proteins and commensal microbes or reactive responses against noxious antigens like those from pathogenic microbes. The intestinal immune system is committed to discriminating antigens that drive tolerance and those destined for reactive inflammatory responses. In a steady state environment both responses lead to immune homeostasis (Figure 1). However, during dysbiosis, the disturbed microbiota may shape the APC signaling towards inflammatory responses that usually predispose to diseases such as IBD (Murai et al., 2009; Abdelouhab et al., 2012; Baker et al., 2012). Restoring normal microbiota profile to such patients treats the diseases due partly to re-shaping the distorted APC signaling during disease. This chapter discusses the APC-microbiota interaction during health and disease. Exploring such a relationship and its outcome could aid designing medication for gut diseases emanating from microbiata disturbances.

Gut Mononuclear Phagocytes

The gut mononuclear phagocytes committed for antigen presentation are mainly macrophages and DCs. Their identification in the gut mucosa has been challenging and there is less consensus regarding the definition, identification and functions of these cells. In brief, both DCs and macrophages express CD11 (e.g., CD11b, CD11c) and major histocompatibility class (MCH)II although these molecules are traditionally used to identify DCs (Figure 2) (Bain and Mowat 2011). Classically, macrophages lack CD11c. However, some express it at low/intermediate levels, making some investigators to group MHCII^{+}CD11b^{+}CD11c^{int} cells as macrophages and not DCs (Denning et al., 2011).

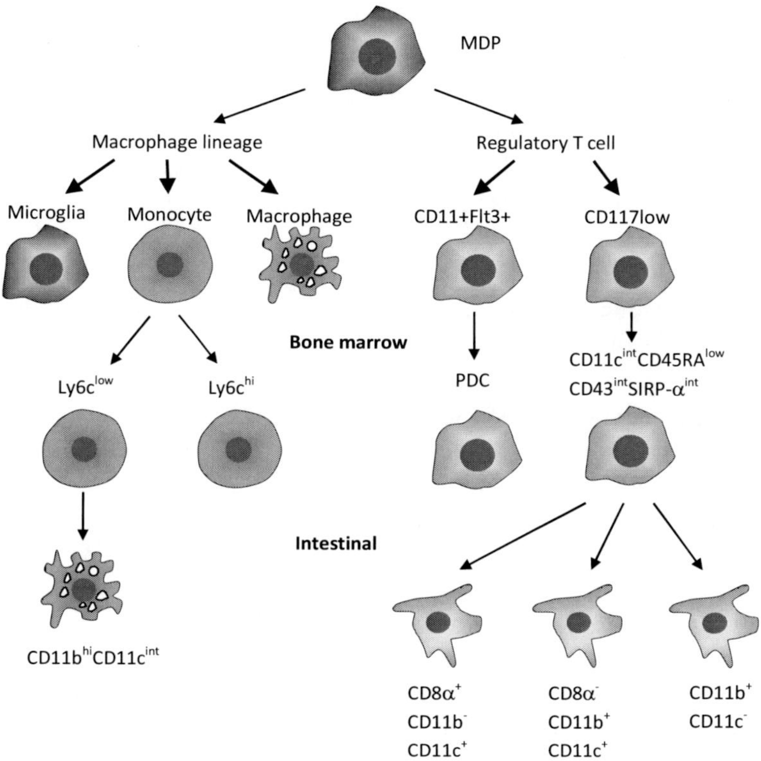

Figure 2. Development and identification of macrophages and dendritic cells. Both macrophages and dendritic cells develop from a common macrophage and dendritic cell progenitor (MDP). Variations in expression of some molecules such as CD11c is useful in discriminating dendritic cells from macrophages. PDC, plasmacytoid dendritic cell.

Expression of another molecule, the fractalkine receptor CX3CR1, has also been used widely to distinguish DCs from macrophages in which case DCs are identified by expression of αE-integrin CD103 and macrophages by CX3CR1 (Bogunovic et al., 2009; Varol et al., 2009; Niess and Adler 2010). It has been shown however that some DCs express intermediate levels of CX3CR1 while some do not express CD103 (Schulz et al., 2009; Bain et al., 2013; Cerovic et al., 2013). This ambiguity can be unraveled from recent findings that have added expression of CD64, CD68, F4/80 and MerTK (Mer tyrosine kinase) as additional criteria to distinguish intestinal DCs and macrophages (Table 1) (Gautier et al., 2012; Tamoutounour et al., 2012; Bain et al., 2013). Thus, in addition to expressing CD11 and MHCII, mononuclear phagocytes expressing CD64, CD68, MerTK and/or F4/80 are identified as macrophages whereas CD64-F4/80$^-$CDc$^+$MHCII$^+$ phagocytes are DCs (Schulz et al., 2009; Bain et al., 2013; Cerovic et al., 2013). In addition, recent finding that all CX3CR1^{hi} mononuclear phagocytes are macrophages despite that CD103$^-$ expressing intermediate levels of CX3CR1 are considered as DCs, is useful in identifying gut macrophages (De Calisto et al., 2012; Bain et al., 2013; Cerovic et al., 2013).

There are several functional differences between macrophages and DCs serving the intestinal immunity. Intestinal macrophages are highly phagocytic cells with abundant foamy cytoplasm (Bain et al., 2013), do not migrate to the mesenteric lymph nodes (MLNs) (Schulz et al., 2009; Cerovic et al., 2013), cannot prime naïve T cells (Schulz et al., 2009), and their development requires colony-stimulating factor-1 receptor (CSF-1R) (MacDonald et al., 2010; Schlitzer et al., 2013). On the contrary, DCs are poorly phagocytic cells, migrate to the MLNs in a CCR7-dependent manner, prime naïve T cells (Schulz et al., 2009; Cerovic et al., 2013), and their development depends on growth factor flt3 ligand (flt3L) (Kim et al., 2014).

Table 1. Identification and differentiation of macrophages and dendritic cells. Macrophages and dendritic cells can be identified and differentiated based on the receptors, functions and molecules required for their development

Criteria	Item	Macrophages	Dendritic cells
Receptors	CD11c	Absent or expressed at intermediate levels	Present
	CX3CR1	Express CX3CR1	• Express CD103 but absent in some DCs • Some DCs express intermediate levels of CX3CR1
	CD64	Present	Absent
	CD68	Present	Absent
	F4/80	Present	Absent
	MerTK	Present	Absent
Functions	Priming naïve T cell	Incapable	Capable
	Phagocytosis	Competent	Poor
	Migration	Immobile	Migrate
Development	Required factor	CSF-1R	FLT3L

The role of microbiota to gut phagocytes has partly been demonstrated by some researchers who identified $CD11c^+$ and $CD11c^-$ cells in intestinal lamina propria (LP) as macrophages that constitutively release high levels of IL-10 in response to the microbiota (Rivollier et al., 2012). In addition, they identified $CD103^+CX3CR1^-CD11b^-$, $CD103^+CX3CR1^-CD11b^+$, and $CD103^-CX3CR1^{int}CD11b^+$ as DCs. These cells came from $Ly6C^{hi}$ monocytes which differentiated into regulatory $CD11c^+$ but not $CD11c^-$ macrophages in non-inflammatory conditions and into pro-inflammatory $CD103^-CX3CR1^{int}CD11b^+$ DCs during colitis. The researchers concluded that the balance of these immunologically antagonistic cell types is dictated by microenvironmental conditions. Indeed, these conditions point to a stable or disrupted microbiota and the consequences thereof (Rivollier et al., 2012).

Other researchers observed a crosstalk between macrophages, DCs and microbiota during antigen presentation to T cells (Mazzini et al., 2014). They found that chemokine receptor $CX3CR1^+$ macrophages take up soluble fed antigens and quickly transfer them to $CD103^+$ DCs in a connexin 43-dependent and membrane transfer mechanisms. Deletion of connexin 43 in these cells affects antigen transfer and fails the $CD103^+$ DC acquisition and presentation of antigens to drive Treg differentiation and to induce tolerance to food antigens. They suggested that this macrophage-DCs crosstalk might be a mechanism by which tolerogenic DCs avoid exposure to the intestinal microbiota. Since both macrophages and DCs are influenced by microbiota, the role of microbiota to this crosstalk could be highly significant

MACROPHAGES

What Are Macrophages?

Gut macrophages are mostly located in the LP of the gut mucosa throughout the entire gastrointestinal tract (Hume et al., 1984). A small population is also present in the smooth muscle layers of the gastrointestinal tract that plays role in regulating intestinal motility (Mikkelsen and Rumessen, 1992; Tajima et al., 2012). The intestinal macrophages form the largest pool of macrophages in the body. They are involved in maintaining microbiota-host homeostasis, intestinal epithelial renewal and protective immunity.

Classically, macrophages are defined as terminally differentiated non-migratory phagocytic cells that are not involved in priming naïve T cells. There is enough evidence however, that besides their phagocytic function, macrophages play essential role in maintaining gut immune tolerance and can mediate inflammatory responses during perturbations (Kelsall 2008; Bain and Mowat 2011). In a steady state gut environment, anti-inflammatory macrophages scavenge bacteria and drive expansion of Treg in the LP. On the contrary, perturbations to the gut due to immune disorders like IBD induce a switch of gut macrophages into pro-inflammatory cells that account for the disease (Kelsall 2008; Bain and Mowat 2011).

Characterization of Intestinal Macrophages

Intestinal macrophages have been characterized into several groups. In the intestine of human patients with IBD, two $CD68^+$ populations of macrophages exist. Firstly, a population that is predominant in a steady-state constituting of $CD14^-$ macrophages. Macrophages in this population do not express receptors for innate response, are hyporesponsive to stimulation by TLR ligands, and do not produce pro-inflammatory cytokines. However, they perform phagocytic and bactericidal activity and express low levels of co-stimulatory molecules CD80, CD86 and CD40 (Smith et al., 2001; Smythies et al., 2005; Mann and Li 2014). The second population is composed of $CD14^+$ macrophages observed to invade the intestinal mucosa during IBD. This population is responsible for driving the disease (Kamada et al., 2008).

In the small intestine of mouse the macrophage population identified composes of $CD11c^-F4/80^+CD11b^+$ cells (Figure 2). This macrophage population expresses IL-10 and drives the differentiation of $Foxp3^+$ Treg cells while suppressing that of Th17 (Denning et al., 2007). In the colon LP of these animals, Rivollier and others (Rivollier et al., 2012) identified $CD11c^+$ and $CD11c^-$ cells as macrophages that constitutively release high levels of IL-10. In non-inflammatory conditions, $CD11c^+$ but not $CD11c^-$ macrophage is produced. It appears that CD11c- may be involved in the inflammatory responses. Other studies identified $CD11c^{-/lo}$F4/80+CD11b+ cells as the mouse colonic macrophages (Platt et al., 2010).

Recent studies are fundamentally grouping gut macrophages as either large population of non-inflammatory resident regulatory $CX3CR1^{hi}$ macrophages or small population of inflammatory $CX3CR1^{int}$ macrophages. The two groups are derived from the same $Ly6C^+CCR2^+$ precursor. Their difference is attributed to different phases of differentiation. Thus, whereas $CX3CR1^{hi}$ macrophages do not respond to TLR stimulation, but produce IL-10 constitutively and are fully differentiated, $CX3CR1^{int}$ macrophages are responsive to TLR and infiltrate the mucosa during inflammation. This infiltration is due to arrest in their differentiation (Bain et al., 2013).

Macrophages and Gut Tolerance

The contribution of macrophages to gut tolerance can be through their constitutive production of anti-inflammatory IL-10, generation and maintenance of Tregs, and suppression of effector Th1, Th2 and Th17 (Figure 1). The cytokine IL-10 produced by $CX3CR1^+$ macrophages drives the expansion and differentiation of $Foxp3^+$ Treg in the intestinal mucosal LP (Hadis et al., 2011). It can also be mediated through their F4/80 molecules since F4/80 knockout mice do not develop tolerance nor antigen-specific $CD8^+$ Tregs after being fed soluble antigen (Lin et al., 2005).

Another mechanism proposed for induction of gut tolerance involves a direct targeting of APC by Treg (Shevach 2009). It has been shown that constitutive surface expression of cytotoxic T lymphocyte antigen (CTLA)-4 enables the interaction with co-stimulatory molecules CD80 and CD86 on macrophages. This interaction leads to down-regulated expression of CD80 and CD86 and limits development of adaptive immune responses (Shevach 2009; Onishi et al., 2008). Animals without CTLA-4 such as knockout mice lack tolerance and develop multi-organ inflammation and premature death (Read et al., 2006; Wing et al., 2008).

Influence of Microbiota on Macrophage Functioning during Health and Disease

The effect of microbiota to the macrophage functioning is depicted during development and differentiation of these cells as well as functioning for tolerance and active immune response. The fact that microbiota can influence development and differentiation of macrophages, is depicted by a recent study by Trapecar and others (2014) in neonatal intestine. These investigators monitored the translocation of nuclear factor kappa B (NF-κB) p65 and signal transducers and activators of transcription (Stat)1 which are among the most important intracellular orchestrators of antimicrobial responses following exposure to *Lactobacillus* spp. They observed that microbiota affects early development of macrophages. Furthermore, macrophages residing the intestine in a steady-state are derived from embryonic precursor cells. They seed the intestinal mucosa and proliferate extensively during the neonatal period. From the weaning time, the microbiota drives a process of replacing these cells by chemokine receptor CCR2-dependent influx of Ly6C^{hi} monocytes that differentiate locally into mature, anti-inflammatory macrophages. This microbiota driven process continues throughout adult life to maintain a normal intestinal macrophage pool and tolerance (Bain et al., 2014).

At steady state, the microbiota maintains tolerance partly by inhibiting CX3CR1^{hi} macrophages from transporting both commensal and pathogenic bacteria from the intestinal lumen to MLNs. However, the trafficking of non-invasive bacteria to the MLNs is resumed during dysbiosis. This transport is in a CCR7-dependent manner and leads to induction of immune reaction mediated by both T cell responses and IgA production (Diehl et al., 2013). The microbiota can also engender immune homeostasis by promoting a crosstalk between innate myeloid and lymphoid cells. This phenomenon depends on the ability of macrophages to sense microbial signals and produce IL-1β that triggers production of granulocyte macrophage colony-stimulating factor (GM-CSF) by retinoic acid-related orphan receptor (RORγt)$^{+}$ innate lymphoid cells (ILCs) (Figure 3). Deficient production of GM-CSF alters mononuclear phagocyte effector functions leading to reduced number of Tregs and impaired tolerance (Mortha et al., 2014). Such scenario predisposes to intestinal diseases like IBD. The microbiota-induced macrophage production of IL-1β also drives differentiation of intestinal Th17 cells by acting directly on IL-1R-expressing T cells. In the absence of IL-1β-IL-1R or MyD88 signaling a selective reduction of intestinal Th17 cells and impaired production of IL-17 and IL-22 occurs. This microbiota-mediated macrophage production of IL-1β is critical for Th17 differentiation and has been suggested to be of therapeutic use in Th17-mediated diseases (Shaw et al., 2012).

The ability of microbiota to shape macrophage production of cytokines has further been observed in experiments involving specific microbiota species. *Lactobacillus reuteri, L. rhamnosus, L. plantarum, Bifidobacterium animalis, B. bifidum, B. longum,* and *B. longum* subsp. *infantis* have been demonstrated to suppress macrophage production of pro-inflammatory TNF-α and IL-1β but increase production of anti-inflammatory cytokines like IL-4 and IL-10 (Figure 4). Both macrophage-shaped responses protect against intestinal lipopolysaccharide (LPS)-induced colitis (Rodes et al., 2013). Under disease conditions, the anti-inflammatory IL-10 produced by intestinal macrophages maintains the expression of Foxp3 on Treg to suppress colitis (Murai et al., 2009). Furthermore, the microbiota negatively regulates macrophage production of pro-inflammatory cytokines via production of IL-10. Normally colonic LP macrophages are primed by microbiota to be unresponsive to LPS in terms of producing pro-inflammatory cytokines but constitutively produce IL-10 to prevent inflammatory reactions (Figure 4). Macrophages from germ-free animals and mice lacking IL-10 or Stat3 tend to have increased levels of LPS-induced TNF-α and IL-6 production (Ueda et al., 2010). By negatively regulating pro-inflammatory cytokines, the microbiota-macrophage interaction maintains intestinal immune homeostasis and could contribute to prevention of different forms of intestinal diseases.

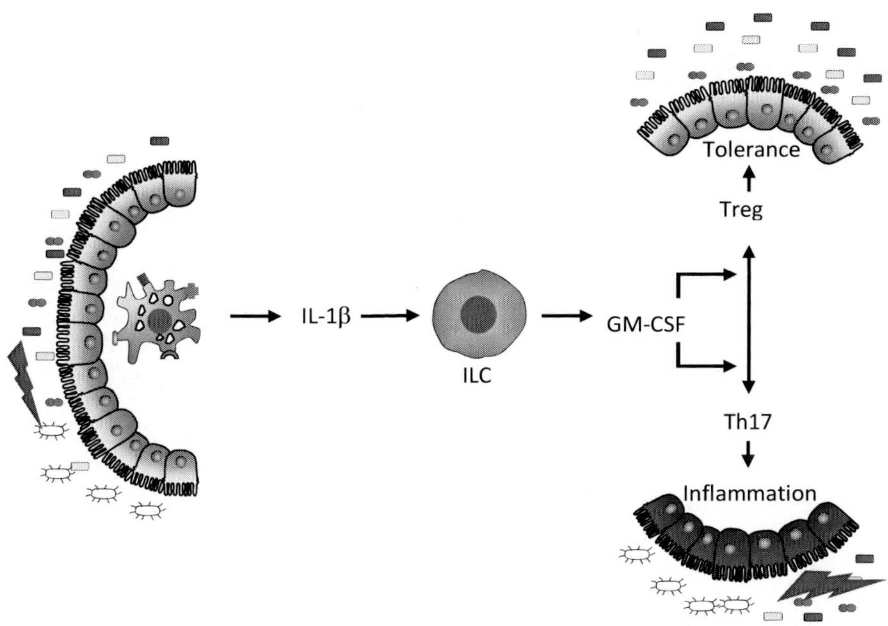

Figure 3. Influence of microbiota on macrophage functioning. Sensing of enteral antigens by macrophages induces production of interleukin (IL)-1β that activates innate lymphoid cell (ILC) to produce GM-CSF (granulocyte-macrophage colony-stimulating factor). In turn, GM-CSF drives regulatory T cell (Treg) to induce tolerance or Th17 to cause inflammation. The tolerogenic or inflammatory responses stem from the ability of macrophages to sense antigens from either balanced microbiota or disrupted microbiota and pathogens respectively.

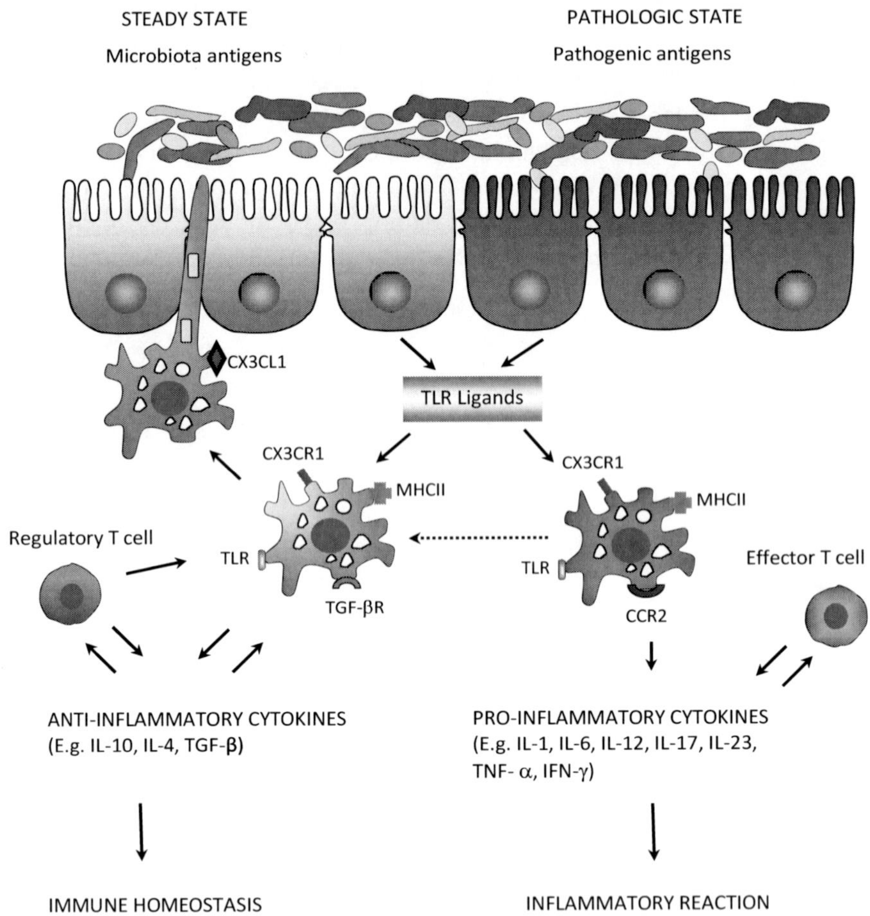

Figure 4. Microbiotal influence on macrophage functioning during health and disease. During intestinal steady state, macrophages sample microbiota antigens, produce anti-inflammatory cytokines, and polarise regulatory T cells to induce immune homeostasis. On the contrary, during infections, macrophages sample pathogenic antigens, produce pro-inflammatory cytokines a nd polarise effector T cells to cause inflammation. IFN, interferon; IL, interleukin; MHC, major histocompatibility class; TGF, transforming growth factor; TLR, toll-like receptor; TNF, tumour necrosis factor.

The shaping of macrophage signaling towards protective direction has been observed to occur during recovery of previously disrupted microbiota. For instance, small bowel resection (SBR) that disrupts colonic microbiota by decreasing the *Firmicutes*, increases the number of macrophages and their pro-inflammatory cytokines IL-1β, IL-6, IL-8, IL-18 and TNF-α in colonic mucosa leading to clinical short bowel syndrome (SBS) (Lapthorne et al., 2013). A similar decrease in *Firmicutes* occurring in mice predisposes the animals to *Citrobacter rodentium* infection (Figure 5). This infection causes acute colitis characterized by increased colonic mucosal macrophages, pro-inflammatory macrophage inflammatory protein (MIP)-2α, inducible nitric oxide synthase (iNOS), IFN-γ, IL-22, and TNF-α expression (Baker et al., 2012). Maneuvers that specifically enrich colonic *Firmicutes* (including increased segmented filamentous bacteria, SFB), and decrease γ-*Proteobacteria*, and those manipulating the microbiota in general suppress macrophage induced pro-inflammatory responses and protect against infectious and chemical colitides (Abdelouhab et al., 2012; Baker et al., 2012).

From the above discussed facts it is obvious that by influencing the development, differentiation and functioning of macrophages, the microbiota confers protective role to the gut through tolerogenic and reactive immune responses. Indeed the microbiota-macrophage interaction is pertinent in driving immune homeostasis under health and disease

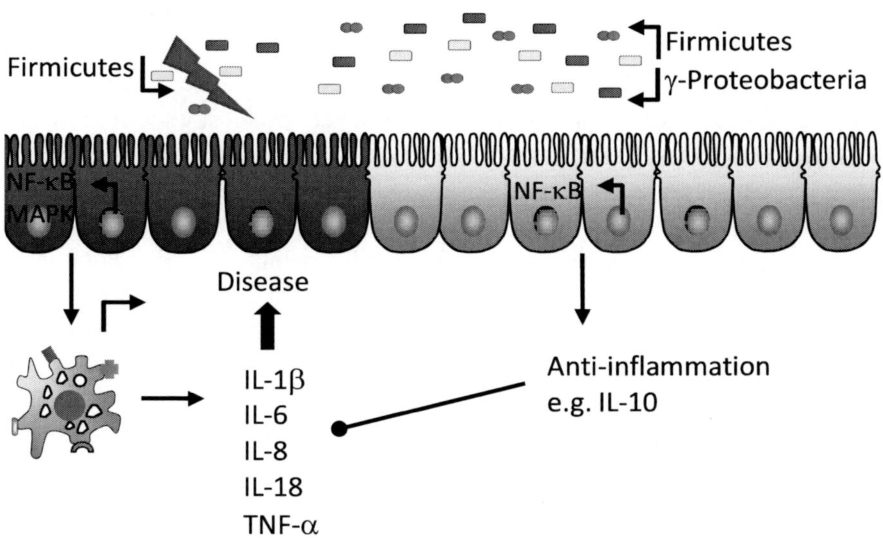

Figure 5. Role of microbiota-macrophage interaction during clinical short bowel syndrome. Disruption of microbiota by decreasing *Firmicutes* increases the number and activity of macrophages leading to clinical short bowel syndrome. Enriching the microbiota with *Firmicutes* or decreasing γ-*Proteobacteria* induces production of anti-inflammatory cytokines that suppress pro-inflammatory response and ameliorates the short bowel syndrome. IL, interleukin; TNF, tumour necrosis factor.

Influence of Microbiota Products on Macrophage Functioning

Apart from the direct effect of microbiota, macrophages can interact with microbiotal fermentation products to maintain gut tolerance and prevent intestinal diseases. Butyrate for instance, renders LP macrophages hyporesponsive to commensal antigens through inhibiting histone deacetylases. This leads to down-regulation of LPS-induced macrophage production of pro-inflammatory mediators, like nitric oxide, IL-6, and IL-12 to curb inflammation and maintain homeostasis (Chang et al., 2014). Kobayashi and others (2012) further demonstrated in germ-free and specific pathogen-free mice that histone deacetylation on IL-12b promoter by histone deacetylase (HDAC)-3 mediates homeostatic effects of IL-10 in macrophages. Butyrate effect can also be mediated through its receptor GPR109A located in the colon. In this case, signaling of GPR109A promotes anti-inflammatory properties in both macrophages and DCs, enabling them to induce differentiation of Treg cells and IL-10-producing T cells. In so doing, the microbiota can suppress colitis and colon cancer in a Gpr109a-dependent manner (Singh et al., 2014). Another study reported that lactic acid producing bacteria and *Clostridium* spp that elevate the levels of short chain fatty acids (SCFAs) (acetate and butyrate) in the hind gut increase the macrophage phagocytic activity and imparts a strong beneficial impact (Geraylou et al., 2012). These studies are indeed, vivid examples of how the microbiota products interact with macrophages to modulate gut immunity by maintaining gut homeostasis and prevent diseases.

DCs

What Are DCs?

DCs are bone marrow derived APCs. Although they are present in small numbers in the intestine, they have a large influence on immune responses. For example, one DC can influence the function of 300 to 1000 T cells (Stagg et al., 2003). Their main functions are acquisition of antigen and stimulation of lymphocytes. Intestinal endocytically active DCs expressing low levels of MHCII and costimulatory molecules like CD40, CD80, and CD86, acquire antigens from microbiota and food proteins in the lumen. These antigens are subsequently presented to lymphocytes to induce immune response. However, at this level, immature DCs whose MHCII expression is low are incapable of stimulating T cells. At times, DCs may undergo maturation and upregulate their expression of MHCII and costimulatory molecules and acquire the ability to activate naïve T cells. When mature DCs encounter antigens from microbial products and/or cytokines like TNF-α transducing danger or tissue damage signals, they migrate to draining lymph nodes

The ability of DCs to activate naïve T cells confers DCs a key role of shaping intestinal immune responses. This involves determining whether tolerance or active immune response should develop from a particular antigen based on whether type 1 or type 2 response predominates. To maintain homeostasis, DCs predominantly drive differentiation of Th2 cells or Treg cells while suppressing differentiation of Th1 (Sato et al., 2003). Furthermore, intestinal DCs drive homing of antigen specific effector cells to LP.

Classification of DCs

DCs are mainly of two classes based on their ability to express the αE-integrin (CD103) or fractalkine receptor (CX3CR1), i.e., $CX3CR1^{-}CD103^{+}$ and $CX3CR1^{+}CD103^{-}$ (Schulz et al., 2009). The $CX3CR1^{-}CD103^{+}$ DCs differentiate from conventional myeloid DC precursors. They typically migrate while transporting microbial antigens from the LP to the MLNs and secondarily to the gut lymphoid tissue (the PPs), to interact with T cells in response to gut antigens. In so doing, they induce expression of CCR9 and α4β7 integrin receptors on naïve T cells which are gut homing receptors pivotal to immunity during homeostasis as well as inflammation. Tolerance towards gut microbiota and food antigens is maintained when DCs sample the antigens and stimulate a balanced differentiation of naïve T cells into either effectors cells (Th1, Th2, Th17) or Treg cells (Tr1, Th3). While IL-2 is responsible for development of Th1, that of Th17 is driven by IL-1 and IL-6. The differentiation into Tr1 and Th3 follows interaction of naïve T cells with immature DCs or the presence of IL-10 and TGF-β (Figure 6). Migration of $CX3CR1^{-}CD103^{+}$ DCs containing alive bacteria to MLNs induces secretory IgA (SIgA)-producing plasma cells (Bar-On et al., 2011; Swiatczak and Rescigno 2012).

The second class of DCs, the $CX3CR1^{+}CD103^{-}$ DCs arises from monocytes through a process mediated by GM-CSF. These DCs are "stationary" and do not typically migrate, have limited ability to activate T cells but restimulate them after challenge, and are involved in sampling of intestinal luminal antigens across the epithelium (Varol et al., 2009; Rescigno 2011; Swiatczak and Rescigno 2012). Both $CX3CR1^{-}CD103^{+}$ and $CX3CR1^{+}CD103^{-}$ DCs are at the interface between the innate and adaptive immune systems.

Location and Functioning of DCs

DCs are located within the GALT in MLNs and PP and are dispersed throughout the subepithelial LP (Varol et al., 2010). Their location enables them to interact, through PRR like TLRs, with microbes arriving to the GALT through M cells. Enteral antigens, particularly from microbiota and food, activate LP plasma cells to produce intestinal SIgA that facilitates bacterial translocation through M cells of PP and ILF. This process sensitizes DCs to sample antigens and decide to tolerate or to mount an immune response to non-self or danger signals. The choice depends on the type and amplitude of the microbial challenge as well as intestinal conditioning of the DCs via micro-environmental signals such as retinoic acid and TGF-β (Rey et al., 2004; Coombes and Powrie 2008; Rescigno 2009; Wang et al., 2009).

The entry of DCs and other lymphocytes into GALT is determined by the interaction between L-selectin receptor (CCR7) and L-selectin ligand (CCL21). It is the role of DCs to direct the lymphocytes location where the antigen is most likely encountered by imprinting tissue specificity. After lymphocytes priming in the lymphoid tissue, the expression of CCR7 and CCL21 adhesion molecules is down regulated and the DCs lose the ability to enter lymphoid tissue. Instead, they gain expression of new adhesion molecules that direct migration to peripheral tissues. Together with $Foxp3^{+}$ Tregs, DCs play key role in maintaining gut tolerance and immune homeostasis by, in part, favoring the induction of Th2 or Treg responses following encounter with microbiotal antigens (Coombes and Maloy 2007). Disruption in this balance results into immune mediated disorders like allergy due to lack of microbial antigen-induced immune deviation from the Th2 to a Th1-cytokine profile that enhances Th2-cell responses to allergens (Purchiaroni et al., 2013).

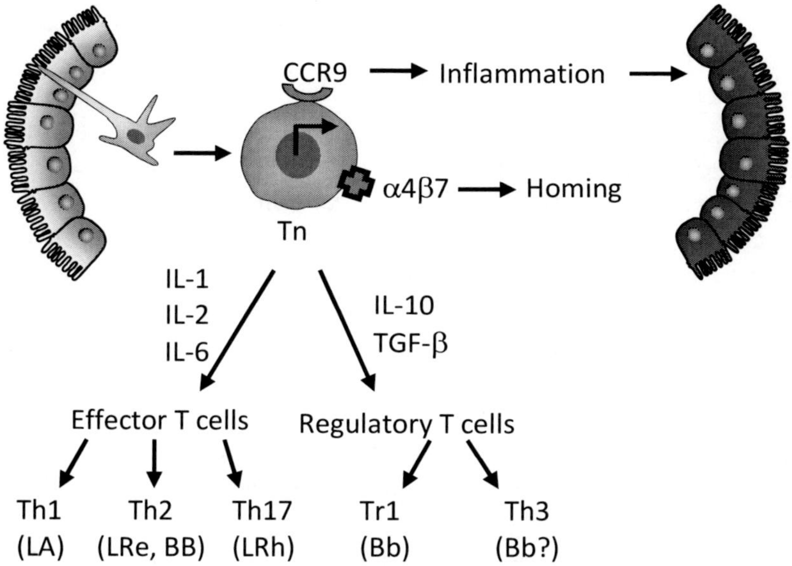

Figure 6. Dendritic cell-mediated microbiotal influence on T cells. Presentation of microbiotal antigens by dendritic cells to naïve T (Tn) cells induces expression of CCR9 and α4β7 integrin receptors on Tn cells for inflammatory and homing responses respectively. The antigen presentation also drives differentiation of effector (e.g., Th1. Th2, Th17) and regulatory (e.g., Tr1, Th3) T cells. Different microbiotal antigens may have different T cell type differentiation. Bb, *Bifidobacterium breve*; BB, *Bifidobacterium bifidum*; IL, interleukin; LA, *Lactobacillus acidophilus*; LRe, *Lactobacillus reuteri*; LRh, *Lactobacillus rhamnosus*; TGF, tumour necrosis factor;

DC Functioning and the Microbiota

The microbiota is central to the modulation of DC functions as well as the immune response. Evidence is mounting on the critical role played by DCs on regulation of gut immunity exhibited by the balance between tolerance to microbiota and active immune response against enteric pathogens. Disruption of this delicate balance often leads to gastrointestinal disorders like IBD. The following sections explore the involvement of microbiota in shaping DC signaling to influence effector cell response.

Influence of Microbiota on Antigen Sampling and Presentation by DCs

Intestinal DCs continually sample luminal antigens and present them to the immune cells in the LP. This can be via M cells of the follicle-associated epithelium of Peyer's patches (PP). The M cells take up luminal antigens and translocate them across the intestinal epithelium to subepithelial dome regions of PP where they deliver them to DCs. In addition, intestinal DCs found at the base of villi and those residing in lymphoid aggregates found in close proximity to the intestinal epithelium also sample luminal antigens (Mowat 2003; Iwasaki, 2007). After sampling, DCs present the antigens directly to GALT or migrate to MLNs to induce immune responses for tolerance or reaction (Niess 2008). Microbiotal uptake by DCs limits bacterial penetration through the intestinal mucosa, neutralizes LPS, and hinders the microbiota from activating the immune system in the LP (Macpherson and Uhr 2004). Furthermore, DCs residing in LP send dendrites across the intestinal epithelium that actively sample luminal antigens from non-invasive bacteria, including microbiota. In so doing, the microbiota induces expression of tight junction proteins that maintain intestinal epithelial barrier integrity and gut immunity (Niess et al., 2005; Rescigno et al., 2001; Farache et al., 2013).

Luminal antigens can also be delivered to underlying LP DCc via goblet cell-associated antigen passages (GAPs) formed by goblet cells in response to acetylcholine (ACh) acting on muscarinic ACh receptor 4. This ACh-induced GAP formation is sensitive to microbiota antigens since Myd88-dependent microbial sensing by colonic goblet cells inhibits the formation of GAPs and the ability of goblet cells to deliver luminal antigens to colonic LP APCs. Disruption of the goblet cell microbial sensing in an intact gut microbiota leads to opening of colonic GAPs, recruitment of neutrophils and APCs and production of inflammatory cytokines (Knoop et al., 2014).

Recent studies have further indicated that antigen sampling and presentation by DCs can be enhanced by specific microbiota species, *Bifidobacterium* species, in IBD patients (Strisciuglio et al., 2014). Similarly, food derived *Lactobacillus* species (*L. plantarum* WCFS1, *L. salivarius* UCC118, and *L. lactis* MG1363) upregulate the activity and numbers of $CD11c^+$ $MHCII^+$ DCs in the immune-sampling PP of healthy mice (Smelt et al., 2013). These facts indicate a potential role of microbiota during disease and health conditions.

Influence of Microbiota on DC-Mediated Tolerance

The microbiota, through pathogen-associated molecular patterns (PAMPs) is recognized by DC TLRs that are highly expressed by DCs. Subsequently, DCs are activated via intracellular signaling molecule TNF receptor associated factor (TRAF)6 to institute gut immune homeostasis. A loss of intestinal mucosa tolerance characterized by development of Th2 cells, eosinophilic enteritis and fibrosis occurs following DC-specific deletion of TRAF6 (Figure 7) (Han et al., 2013). The microbiota can also maintain gut homeostasis by activating DCs to express low levels of MHCII that avoid damage to commensal bacterial (Bell et al., 2001). This could partly be due to the ability of MHCII to drive the microbiota antigen presentation by intestinal DCs to mediate Th17 cell differentiation in the LP and intestinal homeostasis (Goto et al., 2014). The MHCII production profile changes during diseases associated with disruption of microbiota in which case DCs express high levels of MHCII (Sun et al., 2013).

Direct Influence of Microbiota to Functioning of DC and Implication during Disease

The microbiota can drive DCs to produce pro-inflammatory mediators that are responsible for intestinal mucosal surveillance or induce response against noxious agents. Bermudez-Brito and others (2014) have shown that both *Lactobacillus rhamnosus* CNCM I-4036 and its product (cell-free culture supernatant, CFS) induce production of IL-1β, IL-6, IL-8 and IL-12p70 by DCs. The levels of these pro-inflammatory cytokines are higher in DCs treated with the bacterium than in those treated with the CFS. Following *Escherichia coli* infection, the CFS is more effective than the bacterium in reducing the secretion of cytokines. *L. rhamnosus* also induces DCs to produce TGF-β1 and TGF-β2, whereas CFS increases the secretion of TGF-β1 (Bermudez-Brito et al., 2014). In a balanced microbiota, the produced pro-inflammatory cytokines could cater for controlling homeostasis, while in dysbiosis, could drive such diseases like IBD or could be a response to any impending danger in an attempt to protect the gut.

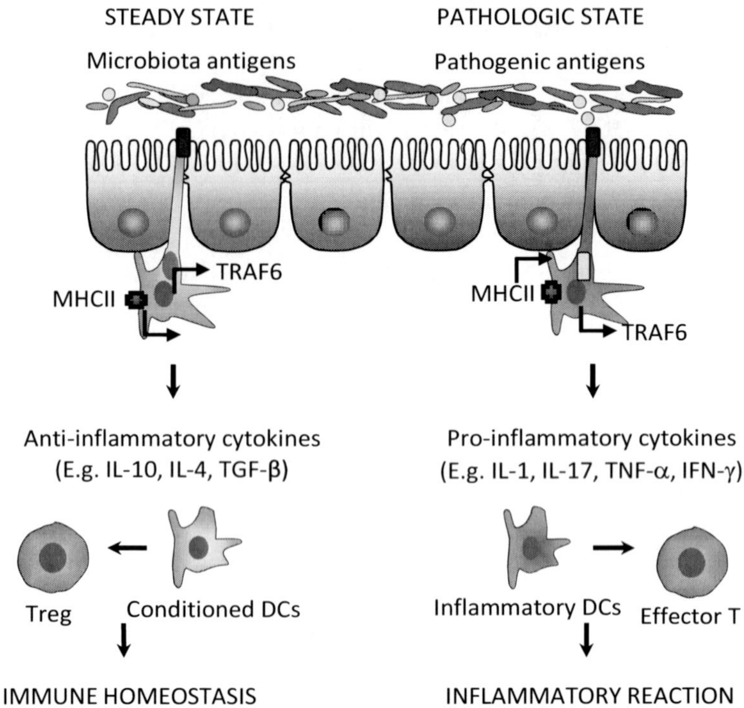

Figure 7. Microbiotal influence on dendritic cell functioning. Dendritic cells sample microbiotal antigens that activate TRAF (tumour necrosis factor (TNF) receptor associated factor)6 but downregulate MHC (major histocompatibility class)II leading to production of anti-inflammatory cytokines that maintain immune homeostasis. During disease, pathogenic antigens activate MHCII and downregulate TRAF6 to cause inflammation. IFN, interferon; IL, interleukin; TGF, transforming growth factor.

Influence of Microbiota on DC-Mediated Induction of T Cells and Implication during Disease

The influence of microbiota to DC-driven T responses has been observed in naïve T, effector Th1, Th2, and Th17 as well as Treg cells involved in gut immunity. Specific microbiota species that have been observed to activate DC to prime naïve T cells include *Lactobacillus acidophilus* that drives DCs to polarize production of Th1, *L. reuteri* and *Bifidobacterium bifidum* for generation of Th2, *L. rhamnosus* that induce production of Th17, and *Bifidobacterium breve* that facilitates production of Tr1 (Figure 6) (Jeon et al., 2012; Dongarrà et al., 2013). The microbiota-T cell specific responses have been earmarked as potential approaches to design therapeutics like probiotics that modulate the gut immune system to overcome diseases.

Polarization of Th1 response by DCs responding to microbiota is depicted from a combination of *L. casei* and TLR3 ligand poly(I:C) that selectively induce DCs to produce substantial amount of IL-6, IL-1β and IL-23 and enhanced levels of IL-12p70. These DCs prime T cells to generate IFN-γ-producing T-bet-positive cells (Th1 cells) without driving a Th17 response. Experiments employing IL-12 monoclonal antibody in DC/T-cell co-cultures show a decreased/inhibited production of IFN-γ and impaired Th1 differentiation (Baba et al., 2009). The *L. casei* plus poly(I:C) is considered an *in vitro* model of viral intestinal infection. As such, the ability to polarise Th1 responses could have protective role in intestinal viral diseases. Besides *L. casei*, *Bifidobacterium infantis* 35624, acting through retinaldehyde dehydrogenase (RALDH) also influences DC signaling by inducing production and increase in the number of DCs which in turn, increases production of Treg $Foxp3^+$ cells but reduce that of Th1 and Th17 in the intestinal LP. The *B. infantis* 35624-induced decrease in Th1 and Th17 reduces the severity of dextran sulphate sodium (DSS)-induced colitis (Konieczna et al., 2013)

Although literature on the microbiota-mediated priming of DC effect to Th2 cells is scant, clear example of this interaction is depicted by the ability of microbiota-stimulated TRAF6 to balance production and function of Treg versus Th2 cells. To achieve this, the microbiota directs DCs to polarize the T cell responses (Han et al., 2013). The significance of this signaling is maintenance of intestinal tolerance. In the absence of TRAF6, the microbiota influences loss of intestinal tolerance manifested by generation of Th2 cells in the LP, eosinophilic enteritis and intestinal fibrosis.

The role of microbiota to drive Th17 production by activating DCs has been described by several researchers. According to Goto and others (2014), commensal SFB sampled by DCs, primes and induces generation of Th17 cells in a MHCII dependent antigen presentation manner. The generated Th17 contributes to intestinal protection and is essential for immunity. Deficiency of MHCII promotes production of Th17 through different pathways independent from SFB while dysregulation of Th17 cells results in autoimmunity. The ability of DCs to polarize Th17 cells is affected by microbial products like bacterial LPS. DCs express acyloxyacyl hydrolase (AOAH) enzyme that inactivates microbiota LPS to polarize and generate Th17 effector cells (Janelsins et al., 2014). Apart from protecting the intestine, the microbiota-DC-Th17 signaling is essential for preventing other gut associated diseases like diabetes mellitus. According to Alam and others (2010), diabetogenic diet disrupts the microbiota profile leading to disturbed gut tolerance to commensals. This causes an increase in production of CD4 T cells, DCs, Th17, and IL-23 and the resulting disease. Feeding of subjects with antidiabetogenic diet induces proliferation of insulin-specific CD4 T cell production and curbs the disease.

Another way by which DCs can shape effector responses is by expressing myeloid C-type lectin receptors (CLRs) that enable them bind to glycan structures present on self or foreign antigens. Clinically, the significance of CLRs stems from their involvement in IBD pathogenesis. Both the macrophage-restricted C-type lectin (MCL) and the DC immunoreceptor (DCIR) bind to intestinal microbiota to modulate production of pro-inflammatory cytokines by these cells and impact subsequent T cell responses. $MCL^{-/-}$ as well as $DCIR^{-/-}$ mice exhibit an increased severity of colitis compared to wild-type counterparts indicating a role for MCL and DCIR in the regulation of intestinal immunity (Hütter et al., 2014)

Effect on Treg

Several studies have demonstrated the ability of microbiota to direct DC-polarization of Treg cells through different ways. Feng and colleagues reported that mucosal DCs express high levels of TLR5 protein in a steady state gut. This expression is downregulated following treatment with various bacterial ligands but promoted by retinoic acid and host stromal cell-derived signals in a TGF-β-independent mechanism. The DC signaling through TLR5 restrains Treg cell generation whereas mice lacking TLR signaling ($TLR5^{-/-}$) have increased $Foxp3^+$ Treg cells in the intestinal LP (Feng et al., 2012). The microbiota can also influence DC-mediated Treg cell functioning via its carbohydrate fermentation products, the SCFAs like butyrate as well as niacin. These chemicals have recently been shown to promote anti-inflammatory activity of DCs by stimulating them to induce differentiation of Treg cells and IL-10-producing T cells through their receptor GPR109A (Singh et al., 2014). The microbiota can also maintain balance between pro- and anti-inflammatory mechanisms through the SCFAs by inhibiting histone deacetylase (HDAC) (Arpaia et al., 2013). The produced SCFAs, at least in part, facilitate extrathymic differentiation of Treg cells in an intronic enhancer CNS1 (conserved non-coding sequence 1, essential for extrathymic Treg-cell differentiation)-dependent manner.

The microbiota-DC interaction can specifically influence Tr1 cell functioning. This is exemplified by a crosstalk between intestinal DCs and *Bifidobacterium breve* designated at inducing development of Tr1. The crosstalk starts with *B. breve* activating intestinal $CD103^+$ DCs to produce IL-10 and IL-27. The produced cytokines drive generation of Tr1 which subsequently produce IL-10 as a potent anti-inflammatory mediator, and express cMaf, IL-21, and Ahr (aryl hydrocarbon receptor) in the large intestine. $CD103^+$ DCs from $IL\text{-}10^{-/-}$, $Tlr2^{-/-}$, and $Myd88^{-/-}$ mice exhibit defective *B. breve*-induced Tr1 cell development and may predispose to intestinal diseases. This interaction is vital in preventing intestinal inflammatory conditions as demonstrated by *B. breve*-mediated amelioration of colitis in immunocompromised mice given naïve T cells from wild type counterparts (Jeon et al., 2012).

EFFECT ON B CELLS

Although the influence of microbiota to B cells is broadly discussed in a separate chapter, it is worth noting that apart from polarizing T cell responses, the microbiota-DCs interaction can also stimulate production of intestinal IgA in a T cell-independent manner but through BAFA and/or APRIL costimulation (Konrad et al., 2006). The produced IgA regulates microbiotal diversity and function as well as intestinal immunity.

CONCLUSION

The intestinal microbiota influences macrophage and DC development, differentiation and functioning for tolerance and active immune response geared at maintaining immune homeostasis. In the absence of microbiota or during dysbiosis, macrophages and DCs drive inflammatory responses leading to diseases that can be deleterious to the host. The microbiota-mediated macrophage and DC protective responses are manifested by the ability of the commensals to shape the effector products of these cells. As a result, the microbiota prevents intestinal diseases that would otherwise develop from activated macrophages and DCs. This phenomenon, as described herein, can further be exploited in order to improve the functioning of microbiota in shaping macrophages and DCs for intestinal immunity. Thus, gaining more insight into the macrophage-/DC-microbiota interaction could aid designing and developing therapeutics against intestinal diseases caused by disruption of microbiota.

REFERENCES

Abdelouhab, K; Rafa, H; Toumi, R; et al. Mucosal intestinal alteration in experimental colitis correlates with nitric oxide production by peritoneal macrophages: effect of probiotics and prebiotics. *Immunopharmacol Immunotoxicol.*, 2012, 34, 590-597.

Alam, C; Valkonen, S; Palagani, V; et al. Inflammatory tendencies and overproduction of IL-17 in the colon of young NOD mice are counteracted with diet change. *Diabetes.*, 2010, 59, 2237-2246.

Amu, S; Saunders, SP; Kronenberg, M; et al. Regulatory B cells prevent and reverse allergic airway inflammation via FoxP3-positive T regulatory cells in a murine model. *J Allergy Clin Immunol.*, 2010, 125, 1114-1124.

Arpaia, N; Campbell, C; Fan, X; et al. Metabolites produced by commensal bacteria promote peripheral regulatory T-cell generation. *Nature.*, 2013, 504, 451-455.

Baba, N; Samson, S; Bourdet-Sicard, R; et al. Selected commensal-related bacteria and Toll-like receptor 3 agonist combinatorial codes synergistically induce interleukin-12 production by dendritic cells to trigger a T helper type 1 polarizing programme. *Immunology.*, 2009, 128(1 Suppl), e523-31.

Bain, CC; Bravo-Blas, A; Scott, CL; et al. Constant replenishment from circulating monocytes maintains the macrophage pool in the intestine of adult mice. *Nat Immunol.*, 2014, In press.

Bain, CC; Mowat, AM. Intestinal macrophages – specialised adaptation to a unique environment. *Eur J Immunol.*, 2011, 41, 2494–2498.

Bain, CC; Scott, CL; Uronen-Hansson, H; et al. Resident and pro-inflammatory macrophages in the colon represent alternative context-dependent fates of the same Ly6Chi monocyte precursors. *Mucosal Immunol.*, 2013, 6, 498-510.

Baker, J; Brown, K; Rajendiran, E; et al. Medicinal lavender modulates the enteric microbiota to protect against Citrobacter rodentium-induced colitis. *Am J Physiol Gastrointest Liver Physiol.*, 2012, 303, G825-836.

Bar-On, L; Birnberg, T; Kim, KW; et al. Dendritic cell-restricted CD80/86 deficiency results in peripheral regulatory T-cell reduction but is not associated with lymphocyte hyperactivation. *Eur J Immunol.*, 2011, 41, 291-298.

Batista, FD; Harwood, NE. The who, how and where of antigen presentation to B cells. *Nat Rev Immunol.*, 2009, 9, 15-27

Bell, SJ; Rigby, R; English, N; et al. Migration and maturation of human colonic dendritic cells. *J Immunol.*, 2001, 166, 4958-4967.

Bermudez-Brito, M; Muñoz-Quezada, S; Gomez-Llorente, C; et al. Lactobacillus rhamnosus and its cell-free culture supernatant differentially modulate inflammatory biomarkers in Escherichia coli-challenged human dendritic cells. *Br J Nutr.*, 2014, 111, 1727-1737.

Bogunovic, M; Ginhoux, F; Helft, J; et al. Origin of the lamina propria dendritic cell network. *Immunity.*, 2009, 31, 513-525.

Cerovic, V; Houston, SA; Scott, CL; et al. Intestinal CD103(-) dendritic cells migrate in lymph and prime effector T cells. *Mucosal Immunol.*, 2013, 6, 104-113

Chang, PV; Hao, L; Offermanns, S; et al. The microbial metabolite butyrate regulates intestinal macrophage function via histone deacetylase inhibition. *Proc Natl Acad Sci U S A.*, 2014, 111, 2247-2252.

Coombes, JL; Maloy, KJ. Control of intestinal homeostasis by regulatory T cells and dendritic cells. *Semin Immunol.*, 2007, 19, 116-126.

Coombes, JL; Powrie, F. Dendritic cells in intestinal immune regulation. *Nat Rev Immunol.*, 2008, 8, 435-446.

De, Calisto, J; Villablanca, EJ; Mora, JR. FcγRI (CD64): an identity card for intestinal macrophages. *Eur J Immunol.*, 2012, 42, 3136-3140.

Denning, TL; Norris, BA; Medina-Contreras, O; et al. Functional specializations of intestinal dendritic cell and macrophage subsets that control Th17 and regulatory T cell responses are dependent on the T cell/APC ratio, source of mouse strain, and regional localization. *J Immunol.*, 2011, 187, 733-747.

Denning, TL; Wang, YC; Patel, SR; et al. Lamina propria macrophages and dendritic cells differentially induce regulatory and interleukin 17-producing T cell responses. *Nat Immunol.*, 2007, 8, 1086-1094.

Diehl, GE; Longman, RS; Zhang, JX; et al. Microbiota restricts trafficking of bacteria to mesenteric lymph nodes by CX(3)CR1(hi) cells. *Nature.*, 2013, 494, 116-120.

Dongarrà, ML; Rizzello, V; Muccio, L; et al. Mucosal immunology and probiotics. *Curr Allergy Asthma Rep.*, 2013, 13, 19-26.

Farache, J; Koren, I; Milo, I; et al. Luminal bacteria recruit CD103+ dendritic cells into the intestinal epithelium to sample bacterial antigens for presentation. *Immunity.*, 2013, 38, 581-595

Feng, T; Cong, Y; Alexander, K; et al. Regulation of Toll-like receptor 5 gene expression and function on mucosal dendritic cells. *PLoS One.*, 2012, 7, e35918.

Fujimoto, K; Karuppuchamy, T; Takemura, N; et al. A new subset of CD103+CD8alpha+ dendritic cells in the small intestine expresses TLR3, TLR7, and TLR9 and induces Th1 response and CTL activity. *J Immunol.*, 2011, 186, 6287-6295.

Gautier, EL; Shay, T; Miller, J; et al. Immunological Genome Consortium. Gene-expression profiles and transcriptional regulatory pathways that underlie the identity and diversity of mouse tissue macrophages. *Nat Immunol.*, 2012, 13, 1118-1128.

Geraylou, Z; Souffreau, C; Rurangwa, E; et al. Effects of arabinoxylan-oligosaccharides (AXOS) on juvenile Siberian sturgeon (Acipenser baerii) performance, immune responses and gastrointestinal microbial community. *Fish Shellfish Immunol.*, 2012, 33, 718-724.

Goto, Y; Panea, C; Nakato, G; et al. Segmented filamentous bacteria antigens presented by intestinal dendritic cells drive mucosal Th17 cell differentiation. *Immunity.*, 2014, 40, 594-607.

Hadis, U; Wahl, B; Schulz, O; et al. Intestinal tolerance requires gut homing and expansion of FoxP3+ regulatory T cells in the lamina propria. *Immunity*, 2011, 34, 237-246.

Han, D; Walsh, MC; Cejas, PJ; et al. Dendritic cell expression of the signaling molecule TRAF6 is critical for gut microbiota-dependent immune tolerance. *Immunity.*, 2013, 38, 1211-1222.

Hume, DA; Perry, VH; Gordon, S. The mononuclear phagocyte system of the mouse defined by immunohistochemical localisation of antigen F4/80: macrophages associated with epithelia. *Anat Rec.*, 1984, 210, 503–512.

Hütter, J; Eriksson, M; Johannssen, T; et al. Role of the C-type lectin receptors MCL and DCIR in experimental colitis. *PLoS One.*, 2014 9, e103281.

Iwasaki, A. Mucosal dendritic cells. *Annu Rev Immunol.*, 2007, 25, 381-418.

Janelsins, BM; Lu, M; Datta, SK. Altered inactivation of commensal LPS due to acyloxyacyl hydrolase deficiency in colonic dendritic cells impairs mucosal Th17 *immunity. Proc Natl Acad Sci U S A.*, 2014, 111, 373-378.

Jeon, SG; Kayama, H; Ueda, Y; et al. Probiotic Bifidobacterium breve induces IL-10-producing Tr1 cells in the colon. *PLoS Pathog.*, 2012, 8, e1002714.

Kamada, N; Hisamatsu, T; Okamoto, S; et al. Unique CD14 intestinal macrophages contribute to the pathogenesis of Crohn disease via IL-23/IFN-gamma axis. *J Clin Invest.*, 2008, 118, 2269-80.

Kelsall, B. Recent progress in understanding the phenotype and function of intestinal dendritic cells and macrophages. *Mucosal immunology.*, 2008, 1, 460–469.

Kim, SW; Choi, SM; Choo, YS; et al. Flt3 ligand induces monocyte proliferation and enhances the function of monocyte-derived dendritic cells in vitro. *J Cell Physiol.*, 2014, In press.

Knoop, KA; McDonald, KG; McCrate, S; McDole, JR; Newberry, RD. Microbial sensing by goblet cells controls immune surveillance of luminal antigens in the colon. *Mucosal Immunol.*, 2014, In press.

Kobayashi, T; Matsuoka, K; Sheikh, SZ; et al. IL-10 regulates IL-12b expression via histone deacetylation: implications for intestinal macrophage homeostasis. *J Immunol.*, 2012, 189, 1792-1799.

Konieczna, P; Ferstl, R; Ziegler, M; et al. Immunomodulation by Bifidobacterium infantis 35624 in the murine lamina propria requires retinoic acid-dependent and independent mechanisms. *PLoS One.*, 2013, 8, e62617.

Konrad, A; Cong, Y; Duck, W; et al. Tight mucosal compartmentation of the murine immune response to antigens of the enteric microbiota. *Gastroenterology.*, 2006, 130, 2050-2059.

Lapthorne, S; Pereira-Fantini, PM; Fouhy, F; et al. Gut microbial diversity is reduced and is associated with colonic inflammation in a piglet model of short bowel syndrome. *Gut Microbes.*, 2013, 4, 212-221.

Lee, JH; Noh, J; Noh, G; et al. Allergen-specific transforming growth factor-β-producing CD19+CD5+ regulatory B-cell (Br3) responses in human late eczematous allergic reactions to cow's milk. *J Interferon Cytokine Res*, 2011, 31, 441-449

Lin, HH; Faunce, DE; Stacey, M; et al. The macrophage F4/80 receptor is required for the induction of antigen-specific efferent regulatory T cells in peripheral tolerance. *J Exp Med 2005*, 201, 1615-1625

MacDonald, KP; Palmer, JS; Cronau, S; et al. An antibody against the colony-stimulating factor 1 receptor depletes the resident subset of monocytes and tissue- and tumor-associated macrophages but does not inhibit inflammation. *Blood.*, 2010, 116, 3955-3963.

Macpherson, AJ; Uhr, T. Induction of protective IgA by intestinal dendritic cells carrying commensal bacteria. *Science.*, 2004, 303, 1662-1665.

Manicassamy, S; Pulendran, B. Retinoic acid-dependent regulation of immune responses by dendritic cells and macrophages. *Semin Immunol.*, 2009, 21, 22–27.

Mann, ER; Li, X. Intestinal antigen-presenting cells in mucosal immune homeostasis: Crosstalk between dendritic cells, macrophages and B-cells. *World J Gastroenterol.*, 2014, 20, 9653-9664

Mann, MK; Maresz, K; Shriver, LP; et al. B cell regulation of CD4+CD25+ T regulatory cells and IL-10 via B7 is essential for recovery from experimental autoimmune encephalomyelitis. J Immunol 2007, 178, 3447-3456

Mazzini, E; Massimiliano, L; Penna, G; et al. Oral tolerance can be established via gap junction transfer of fed antigens from $CX3CR1^+$ macrophages to $CD103^+$ dendritic cells. *Immunity.*, 2014, 40, 248-261.

Mikkelsen, HB; Rumessen, JJ. Characterization of macrophage-like cells in the external layers of human small and large intestine. *Cell Tissue Res*, 1992, 270, 273–279.

Mortha, A; Chudnovskiy, A; Hashimoto, D; et al. Microbiota-dependent crosstalk between macrophages and ILC3 promotes intestinal homeostasis. *Science.*, 2014, 343, 1249288.

Mowat, AM. Anatomical basis of tolerance and immunity to intestinal antigens. *Nat. Rev. Immunol.*, 2003, 3, 331–341.

Murai, M; Turovskaya, O; Kim, G; et al. Interleukin 10 acts on regulatory T cells to maintain expression of the transcription factor Foxp3 and suppressive function in mice with colitis. *Nat Immunol.*, 2009, 10, 1178-1184.

Niess, JH; Adler, G. Enteric flora expands gut lamina propria CX3CR1+ dendritic cells supporting inflammatory immune responses under normal and inflammatory conditions. *J Immunol.*, 2010, 184, 2026–2037.

Niess, JH; Brand, S; Gu, X; et al. CX3CR1- mediated dendritic cell access to the intestinal lumen and bacterial clearance. Science 2005, 307, 254–258.

Niess, JH. Role of mucosal dendritic cells in inflammatory bowel disease. World J Gastroenterol., 2008, 14, 5138–5148.

Onishi, Y; Fehervari, Z; Yamaguchi, T; et al. Foxp3+ natural regulatory T cells preferentially form aggregates on dendritic cells in vitro and actively inhibit their maturation. *Proc Natl Acad Sci U S A.*, 2008, 105, 10113-10118.

Platt, AM; Bain, CC; Bordon, Y; et al. An independent subset of TLR expressing CCR2-dependent macrophages promotes colonic inflammation. *J Immunol.*, 2010, 184, 6843-6854.

Purchiaroni, F; Tortora, A; Gabrielli, M; et al. The role of intestinal microbiota and the immune system. Eur Rev Med Pharmacol Sci., 2013, 17, 323-333.

Read, S; Greenwald, R; Izcue, A; Robinson, N; Mandelbrot, D; Francisco, L, Sharpe, AH; Powrie, F. Blockade of CTLA-4 on CD4+CD25+ regulatory T cells abrogates their function in vivo. *J Immunol.*, 2006 Oct 1, 177(7), 4376-83.

Rescigno, M; Urbano, M; Valzasina, B; et al. Dendritic cells express tight junction proteins and penetrate gut epithelial monolayers to sample bacteria. *Nat Immunol.*, 2001, 2, 361-367.

Rescigno, M. Before they were gut dendritic cells. *Immunity.*, 2009, 31, 454-456.

Rescigno, M. Dendritic cells in bacteria handling in the gut. *J Leukoc Biol.*, 2011, 90, 669-672.

Rey, J; Garin, N; Spertini, F; et al. Targeting of secretory IgA to Peyer's patch dendritic and T cells after transport by intestinal M cells. *J Immunol.*, 2004, 172, 3026-3033.

Rivollier, A; He, J; Kole, A; et al. Inflammation switches the differentiation program of Ly6Chi monocytes from antiinflammatory macrophages to inflammatory dendritic cells in the colon. *J Exp Med.*, 2012, 209, 139-155.

Rodes, L; Khan, A; Paul, A; et al. Effect of probiotics Lactobacillus and Bifidobacterium on gut-derived lipopolysaccharides and inflammatory cytokines: an in vitro study using a human colonic microbiota model. *J Microbiol Biotechnol.*, 2013, 23, 518-526.

Sato, A; Hashiguchi, M; Toda, E; et al. CD11b+ Peyer's patch dendritic cells secrete IL-6 and induce IgA secretion from naive B cells. *J Immunol.*, 2003, 171, 3684-3690.

Schlitzer, A; McGovern, N; Teo, P; et al. IRF4 transcription factor-dependent CD11b+ dendritic cells in human and mouse control mucosal IL-17 cytokine responses. *Immunity.*, 2013, 38, 970-983.

Schulz, O; Jaensson, E; Persson, EK; et al. Intestinal CD103+, but not CX3CR1+, antigen sampling cells migrate in lymph and serve classical dendritic cell functions. *J Exp Med.*, 2009, 206, 3101-3114.

Shaw, MH; Kamada, N; Kim, YG; et al. Microbiota-induced IL-1β, but not IL-6, is critical for the development of steady-state TH17 cells in the intestine. *J Exp Med.*, 2012, 209, 251-258.

Shevach, EM. Mechanisms of foxp3+ T regulatory cell-mediated suppression. *Immunity.*, 2009, 30, 636-645.

Singh, N; Gurav, A; Sivaprakasam, S; et al. Activation of Gpr109a, receptor for niacin and the commensal metabolite butyrate, suppresses colonic inflammation and carcinogenesis. *Immunity.*, 2014, 40, 128-139.

Smelt, MJ; de, Haan, BJ; Bron, PA; et al. Probiotics can generate FoxP3 T-cell responses in the small intestine and simultaneously inducing CD4 and CD8 T cell activation in the large intestine. *PLoS One.*, 2013, 8, e68952.

Smith, PD; Smythies, LE; Mosteller-Barnum, M; et al. Intestinal macrophages lack CD14 and CD89 and consequently are down-regulated for LPS- and IgA-mediated activities. *J Immunol.*, 2001, 167, 2651-2656.

Smythies, LE; Sellers, M; Clements, RH; et al. Human intestinal macrophages display profound inflammatory anergy despite avid phagocytic and bacteriocidal activity. *J Clin Invest.*, 2005, 115, 66-75.

Stagg, AJ; Hart, AL; Knight, SC; et al. The dendritic cell: its role in intestinal inflammation and relationship with gut bacteria. *Gut.*, 2003, 52, 1522-1529.

Steinman, RM. Decisions about dendritic cells: past, present, and future. *Annu Rev Immunol.*, 2012, 30, 1-22.

Strisciuglio, C; Miele, E; Giugliano, FP; et al. Probiotic bacteria enhance antigen sampling and processing by dendritic cells in pediatric IBD. European Crohn's and Colitis Organisation – ECCO, P031, 2014.

Sun, D; Yang, X; Zhao, X; et al. [Alterations in intestinal microflora balance induce maturity and increase the expressions of TLR2 and TLR4 of dendritic cells in mouse lung]. *Xi Bao Yu Fen Zi Mian Yi Xue Za Zhi.*, 2013, 29, 923-926.

Swiatczak, B; Rescigno, M. How the interplay between antigen presenting cells and microbiota tunes host immune responses in the gut. *Semin Immunol.*, 2012, 24, 43-49.

Swiatczak, B; Rescigno, M. How the interplay between antigen presenting cells and microbiota tunes host immune responses in the gut. *Semin Immunol.*, 2012, 24, 43–49.

Tajima, T; Murata, T; Aritake, K; et al. EP2 and EP4 receptors on muscularis resident macrophages mediate LPS-induced intestinal dysmotility via iNOS upregulation through cAMP/ERK signals. *Am J Physiol Gastrointest Liver Physiol.*, 2012, 302, G524-534.

Tamoutounour, S; Henri, S; Lelouard, H; et al. CD64 distinguishes macrophages from dendritic cells in the gut and reveals the Th1-inducing role of mesenteric lymph node macrophages during colitis. *Eur J Immunol.*, 2012, 42, 3150-3166.

Trapecar, M; Goropevsek, A; Gorenjak, M; et al. A co-culture model of the developing small intestine offers new insight in the early immunomodulation of enterocytes and macrophages by Lactobacillus spp. Through STAT1 and NF-kB p65 translocation. *PLoS One.*, 2014, 9, e86297.

Ueda, Y; Kayama, H; Jeon, SG; et al. Commensal microbiota induce LPS hyporesponsiveness in colonic macrophages via the production of IL-10. *Int Immunol.*, 2010, 22, 953-962.

Varol, C; Vallon-Eberhard, A; Elinav, E; et al. Intestinal lamina propria dendritic cell subsets have different origin and functions. *Immunity.*, 2009, 31, 502-512.

Wang, J; Huizinga, TW; Toes, RE. De novo generation and enhanced suppression of human CD4+CD25+ regulatory T cells by retinoic acid. *J Immunol.*, 2009, 183(6), 4119-4126.

Wing, K; Onishi, Y; Prieto-Martin, P; et al. CTLA-4 control over Foxp3+ regulatory T cell function. *Science.*, 2008, 322, 271-275.

Chapter 4

MICROBIOTA AND FUNCTIONING OF INTESTINAL HUMORAL IMMUNITY

ABSTRACT

Intestinal humoral immune system is the major form of adaptive immunity in the intestine. It comprises about two-third of the total body immunoglobulin (Ig) population and 10^6 lymphocytes/g tissue that mediate its responses. Most of the intestinal humoral immune system functions are mediated by IgA and to less extent IgG and IgM secreted by B lymphocytes and plasma cells into the lumen. The B lymphocytes are mainly found in the gut-associated lymphoid tissue (GALT) where inductive and effector sites driving humoral immune response are located. The microbiota facilitates most, if not all, of the humoral immune functions. This is depicted by the ability of the microbiota to drive development and diversity of GALT as well as the resulting immune responses. Whereas the influence of a balanced microbiota favors tolerance to non harmful antigens and immune response against noxious antigens and generates immune homeostasis, disrupted microbiota leads to impaired immunity and disease. Maneuvers that rectify the microbiotal imbalances correct the disrupted microbiota-mediated humoral responses, cure diseases and restore immune homeostasis. Herein, the contribution of microbiota to the intestinal humoral immunity during health and disease is described.

Introduction

In healthy individuals, the ingesta transit time from mouth to anus ranges between 55 and 72 hours, of which 4–6 hours is from the mouth to the cecum and 54–56 hours is in the colon (Cummings et al., 1992). The short transit time through the small intestine does not allow bacterial growth, whereas, in the colon, the much longer transit time contributes significantly to the multiplication of bacteria that reach considerable population levels of up to 1×10^{12} bacterial cells per gram of human colonic content (Garrett et al., 2010; Carvalho et al., 2012). This number exceeds that of human cells by 10 folds, alluding to a significant contribution of microbiota to host immunity. Despite of variable data, the intestinal microbiota population is constituted by 6-10 phyla and approximately up to 5,000 distinct species of bacteria (Garrett et al., 2010; Carvalho et al., 2012). They include *Firmicutes*, *Bacteroidetes*, *Actinobacteria*, *Proteobacteria,* and *Verrucomicrobia* (Tap et al., 2009). The predominant genera are *Faecalibacterium*, *Ruminococcus*, *Eubacterium*, *Dorea*, *Bacteroides*, *Alistipes* and *Bifidobacterium* (Tap et al., 2009).

The intestinal humoral immune system is the major form of adaptive immunity in the intestine. It is directed at microbes in the lumen to prevent commensals and pathogens from colonizing and invading the host through the mucosal epithelial barrier. The significance of this immune system is depicted by the fact that the intestine contains about 60% of the total immunoglobulins (Ig's) and more than 10^6 lymphocytes/g tissue (Salminen et al., 1998). Its functions are mostly mediated by IgA and to a lesser extent IgG and IgM secreted into the intestinal lumen by B lymphocytes or their terminally differentiated plasma cells. The intestinal humoral immune system can tolerate dietary antigens and the gut colonizing bacteria (Hapfelmeier et al., 2010; Pabst 2012). It also recognizes and rejects enteropathogenic microorganisms that may challenge the body's defense.

In the past decade, many studies have explored the contribution of microbiota to the intestinal humoral immunity. The insight gained from these studies indicates that the microbiota is pivotal to the intestinal humoral immunity. Some of these studies have clearly shown that disruption of microbiota balance often leads to disorders related to impaired humoral immunity. For instance, the lack of microbiota in germ-free animals leads to poor formation of spleens, hypoplastic Peyer's patches (PP), decreased number of mature isolated lymphoid follicles (ILF), decreased number of IgA-producing plasma cells as well as the levels of IgA and IgG, irregularities in cytokine levels and profiles, and impaired generation of oral tolerance

(Sekirov et al., 2010). In addition, disruption of microbiota leads to diseases associated with impaired humoral immunity. Correcting the microbiotal imbalances cures the disorders (Brandtzaeg 2013). These defects are clear indications of the importance of the microbiota in humoral intestinal immunity right from the development of the immune system to the operationalization. It is therefore important to explore the microbiota-intestinal humoral immune interaction during gut health and disease so as to learn the possible interventions that can treat immune-mediated diseases. This chapter explores recent findings on the contribution of the microbiota to the functioning of the intestinal humoral immune system in fostering the intestinal immunity. The knowledge gained herein might assist in designing appropriate approaches to manage immune mediated disorders, particularly those resulting from impaired intestinal humoral immunity due to disruption of the microbiota.

Composition of the Intestinal Humoral Immune System

Gut-Associated Lymphoid Tissue, GALT

The intestinal humoral immune system is part of lymphoid immune cells manifested as a complex of immune responses from intestinal epithelium and gut-associated lymphoid tissue (GALT). GALT, which contains up to 30% of the lymphocytes in the body, composes of PP, ILF, intra-epithelial lymphocytes (IEL), lamina propria (LP), mesenteric lymph nodes (MLN), and cryptopatches (CP) (Rescigno 2010). Whereas the IEL and LP are GALT's effector sites, MLN, PP, ILF, and CP serve as inductive sites (Fagarasan et al., 2010). The effector and inductive sites are linked by blood and lymph vessels (Figure 1). The hallmark of organized GALT is the lymphoid follicles, well exemplified by the PP and MLN which are organized intestinal lymphoid follicles. It is in MLN and PP where the responses of adaptive immunity are particularly imprinted.

PPs are mainly found in the distal ileum. They have germinal centers containing naïve B cells, follicular dendritic cells, and T cell rich areas. PPs are lymphoid follicles covered by follicle associated epithelium which contains M cells. The latter are specialized epithelial cells designated for sampling luminal antigens directly into the PP to trigger active or tolerogenic immune response (Locke et al., 2006; Johansson-Lindbom and Agace 2007).

The germinal centers are surrounded by IgM- and IgD-expressing naïve follicular B cells (Figure 1). Between the follicles and the overlying epithelium is an area called the dome that contains B and T lymphocytes, dendritic cells (DCs), and macrophages. In addition, T-cells are found between the follicles in parafollicular areas. The PPs develop in the small intestine during fetal life independently of gut colonization by microbiota and constitute the most prominent IgA inductive site in the GALT (Fagarasan et al., 2010).

The ILF are barrel-shaped, single-domed, mononuclear lymphoid aggregates located throughout the surface of the small intestine and the colon in the antimesenteric wall (Schenk and Mueller 2008). They develop after birth in response to microbiota (Fagarasan et al., 2010). They resemble PP by having an overlying follicle associated epithelium containing M cells, germinal centers and segregated B and T cell areas. Their function is also more or less similar to that of PP.

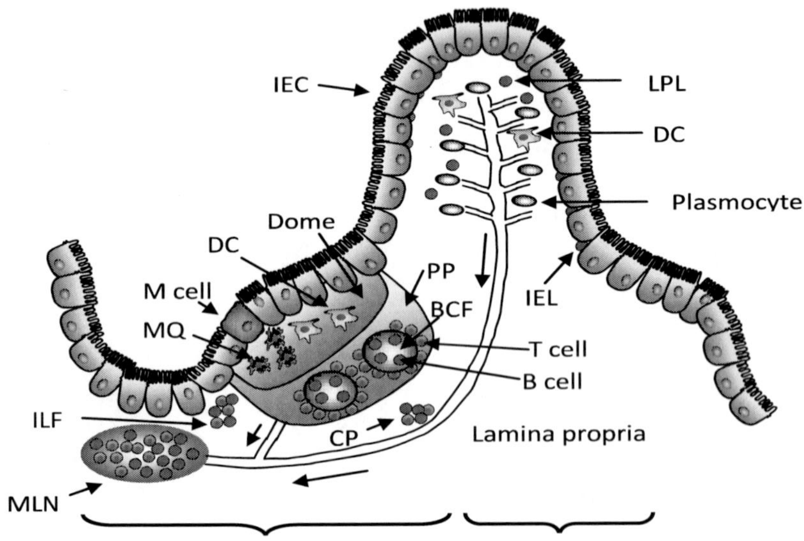

Figure 1. Components of gut-associated lymphoid tissue. GALT (gut-associated lymphoid tissue) composes of effector (IEL and LP) and inductive (MLN, PP, ILF, and CP) sites. Antigens are mainly sampled at effector sites and transported to inductive sites for further processing and execution of adaptive responses. The microbiota influences the development, expansion and functioning of GALT components. BCF, B cell follicle; CP, cryptopatch; DC, dendritic cell; IEC, intestinal epithelial cells; IEL, interepithelial lymphocyte; ILF, isolated lymphoid follicle; LPL, lamina propria lymphocyte; MLN, mesenteric lymph node; MQ, macrophage; PP, Peyer's patch.

The IEL are distinct intestinal immune cell populations. They are T lymphocytes involved mainly in innate immunity and some cytotoxic and regulatory activities necessary for tolerance (Strowig et al., 2012). Some of the T cells such as CD8 lymphocytes migrate to the tip of the villous to become IELs.

As a distinct intestinal immune compartment, the LP is the primary residence of the major components of the adaptive immune system of the gut. It contains B lymphocytes and plasma cells, most of which (about 70-90%) produce IgA that is secreted into the intestinal lumen to prevent epithelial colonization by pathogens and inhibit penetration of harmful foreign material (Mowat and Vinney 1997). It also contains αβ-TCR (T cell receptor) $CD4^+$ and $CD8^+$ effector T cells, T regulatory (Treg) cells, macrophages and DCs (Voss et al., 2006; Vaishnava et al., 2008; Clarke et al., 2010).

MLNs form an organized intestinal lymphoid tissue that filters the mesenteric lymph vessels by collecting intestinal lymph-borne antigens. They develop during fetal life and receive antigens from PPs via afferent lymphatics (Fagarasan et al., 2010).

The MLNs consist of B and T cell areas in which B cells differentiate into dimeric IgA–secreting plasma cells and both effector and Treg cells develop. In addition, MLN contain macrophages serving an antigen presentation to trigger immune response for various purposes (Figure 1). They are sites of differentiation of effector and regulatory lymphocytes that home back to the LP. Upon encounter with antigens presented by antigen presenting cells (APC) (especially DCs) from LP, the MLNs recognise and activate naïve T cells to institute adaptive immunity and tolerance (Hugot et al., 2001; Xavier and Podolsky 2007).

The intestinal CPs are small lymphoid aggregates found in the LP adjacent to intestinal crypts and surrounded by DCs. They are immature lymphocyte-like cells involved in the formation of ILF (Kunkel et al., 2003; Izcue et al., 2009). CPs develop progenitor T cells for extrathymic descendants that migrate to the IEL compartment.

B Cells

B cells in GALT, especially the LP differentiate into plasma cells and produce antibodies (mainly IgA). The B cells include several phenotypically and functionally different subgroups.

The major B cell population during the first years of life is $CD5^+$ B cells, after which they decrease in numbers (Hannet et al., 1992). The $CD5^+$ B cells may contribute to a first line of defense against bacterial infections since they have fewer somatic hypermutations than other B cells such as CD52 and predominantly produce low affinity polyreactive IgM antibodies that cross-react with bacterial antigens, including LPS (Mackenzie et al., 1991; Brezinschek et al., 1997). In mice, the expression of CD5 B cells identifies the specific B cell linage termed B1 (Stall et al., 1996).

The intestinal LP contains IgM^+ B cells that may function as a local precursor of IgA producing plasma cells (Fagarasan et al., 2001). According to Suzuki and others (2005), these IgM^+ precursors are of two categories. The first group includes naïve B cells that migrate from the bone marrow to the intestine in response to chemotactic signals generated by intestinal stromal cells through a lymphotoxin-mediated nuclear factor kappa B (NF-κB)-inducing kinase (NIK)-dependent pathway. The second group comprises gut experienced IgM^+ B cells that migrate from PP to the intestinal LP independent of stromal signals (Suzuki et al., 2005). Furthermore, the intestinal LP of normal but not activation-induced cytidine deaminase (AID)-deficient mice also contains IgA^+ B cells, indicating that resident IgM^+ B cells may switch to IgA-producing plasma cells in situ (Fagarasan et al., 2001). The active IgM to IgA class switching is a well reported phenomenon that is also present in the human intestinal LP (He et al., 2007).

Immunoglobulins

The intestinal humoral immunity is dominated by production of IgA and to a lesser extent IgG and IgM antibodies in the GALT (Corthesy 2013). The produced antibodies are transported across the mucosal epithelium into the intestinal lumen for functioning. Studies have shown that prior to this transportation, monomeric IgA antibodies dimerize by interacting with a small polypeptide called joining (J) chain (Figure 2). The resulting IgA dimers recognize polymeric immunoglobulin receptor (pIgR) located on the basolateral surface of the IECs (Mestecky and McGhee 1987). Subsequently, the pIgR transports the IgA dimers across IECs by transcytosis and facilitates its release as secretory IgA (SIgA) onto the surface of the gut (Strugnell and Wijburg 2010).

The SIgA is finally anchored to mucus to elicit its protection through binding of the antibodies to the mucus layer that separates commensal bacteria from the apical surface of intestinal epithelial cells (IECs) (Johansson et al., 2013). Within the mucus, the antibodies bind to microbes and toxins and neutralize them to inhibit the binding of microbes and toxins to IECs (Phalipon et al., 2002).

The commitment of IgA in maintaining intestinal humoral immunity is exhibited by the ability of IgA-secreting cells to stay in gastrointestinal tract or home back to the intestinal LP. They may reside as plasma cells after homing back if they happen to enter the systemic circulation. The homing back is due to imprinting of IgA producing B cells with gut-homing properties via induction of α4β7 molecule by retinoic acid which is released by DCs from PPs (Mora et al., 2009).

The produced α4β7 binds mucosal addressin cell-adhesion molecule-1 (MadCAM-1) on gut endothelial venules. In addition, retinoic acid induces B-cell expression of a chemokine receptor CCR9 that binds CCL25 from IECs (Figure 2). It is the B cells' response to CCL25 that makes the PP-derived IgA^{+} $\alpha4\beta7^{+}$ $CCR9^{+}$ B cells migrate to the intestinal LP (Mora et al., 2009).

To maintain the abundance of IgA in the intestinal mucosal, B cells in GALT perform selective induction of IgA isotype switching. The end result is preferential production of IgA-producing B cells in the GALT. This isotype switching occurs either through T-dependent or -independent mechanisms. Both mechanisms are driven by cytokines such as transforming growth factor (TGF)-β and tumor necrosis factor family proteins like APRIL and several membrane proteins on other cell types that bind to receptors (e.g., TACI) on B cells.

The functions of SIgA and possibly IgM and IgG in the intestine are to maintain the beneficial non-pathogenic microbiota and neutralize the action of pathogens. This can be achieved by binding the antigen to the variable region of the Igs. This binding blocks certain bacterial epitopes to prevent the adhesion of commensal bacteria with the apical surface of IECs (Strugnell and Wijburg 2010). It has also been shown that SIgA can limit the microbial motility through glycans associated with the short chain (SC) and constant region a (Ca) of IgA. The SIgA also blocks the functioning of microbes and toxins inside the IECs (Strugnell and Wijburg 2010).

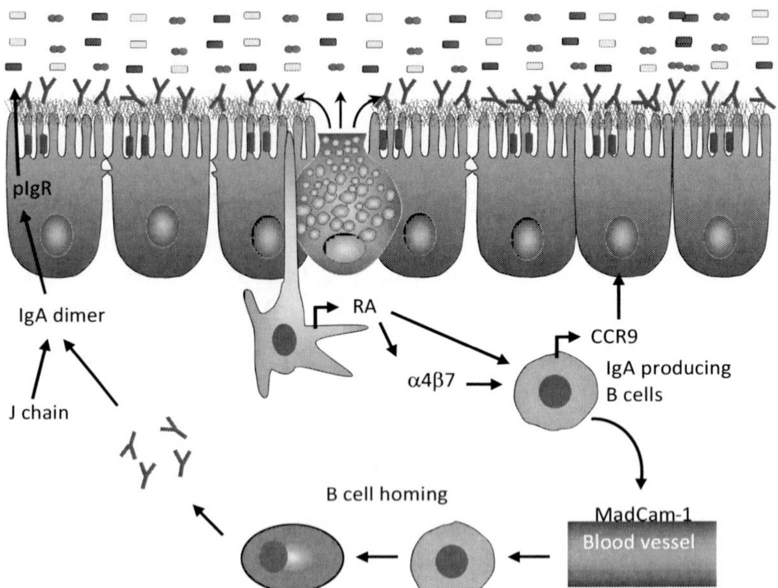

Figure 2. Influence of microbiota on intestinal IgA production. Microbiotal sampling by dendritic cells induces expression of retinoid acid (RA) that induces B-cell homing to produce immunoglobulin (Ig)A. This process is mediated by α4β7 that binds to mucosal addressin cell-adhesion molecule (MadCAM)-1 on gut endothelial venules. The produced IgA dimerizes with J chain, binds to polymeric immunoglobulin receptor (pIgR) on IEC basolateral surface, transported across the IEC and finally secreted onto intestinal apical surface. The secreted IgA regulates commensal profile in the intestinal lumen for health.

Contribution of the Microbiota to the Intestinal Humoral Immunity

Effect on Development, Diversity and Responses

The contribution of microbiota to the intestinal humoral immune system has been a focus of interest in recent years. Mounting evidence shows that it influences the development and regulation of the host's GALT to modulate the humoral immunity (Imaoka et al., 1996; Williams et al., 2006; Bouskra et al., 2008). In germ-free animals for instance, GALT is immature and has reduced number and size. The MLN, PP, LP $CD4^+$ T cells, IgA producing B cells, IEL, and ILF of these animals are also reduced (Imaoka et al., 1996; Williams et al., 2006; Bouskra et al., 2008). Introduction of microbiota in these animals stimulates and promotes the development, expansion and function of the immune system. This is due to the ability of microbiota to drive the expansion of B and T cells in PP and MLN (Figure 3). The larger PP and MLN following colonization with bacteria produce germinal centers that foster the cognate interaction of B cells with $CD4^+$ T cells (Fagarasan et al., 2010). Indeed, follicles from PPs in adult individuals always show prominent germinal centers because of the continuous stimulation of B cells by luminal antigens (Fagarasan et al., 2010).

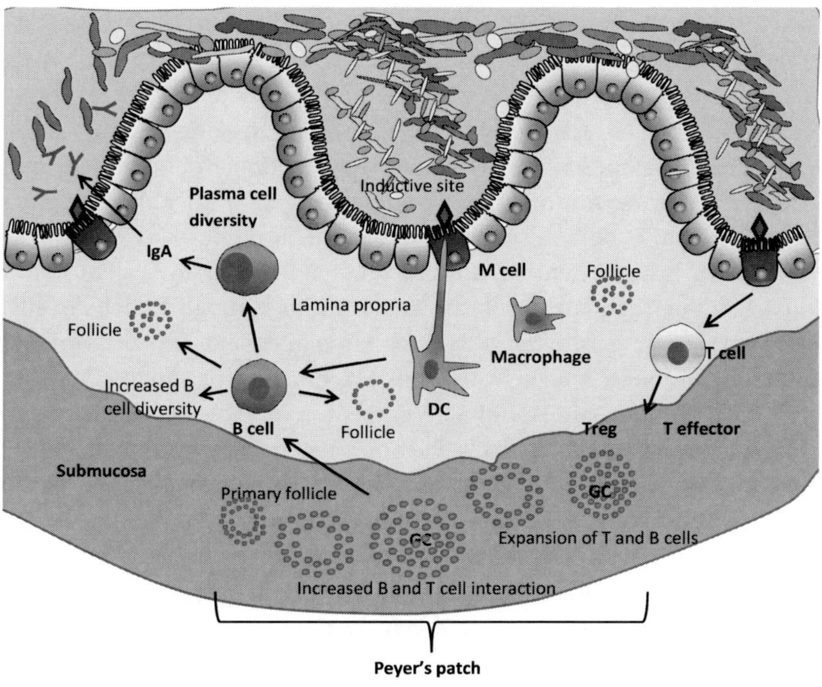

Figure 3. Microbiotal induction of adaptive immune system. The microbiota can 'strike' inductive site through M-cell that samples antigens to dendritic cells or macrophage in lamina propria. This signal is sent to effector site, in this case the Peyer's patch. This brings about development of B cells exemplified by expanded germinal centers (GC) and increased B and plasma cell diversity. The B cells produce immunoglobulin (Ig)A or IgM that is secreted to the lumen for immunity. Sampling of the microbiota antigen by M cells also trigers T cells within the lamina propria that subsequently induce activation of both effector and regulatory T cells for homeostasis and immunity.

The effect of microbiota is also evidenced in its influence on diversity of IgA clones. Normally, the intestinal IgA repertoire is composed of high- and low-frequency clones. Whereas the high frequency clones are presumed to recognize highly prevalent and stable components of the microbiota, the low frequency ones reflect adaptive adjustments to minor changes in the microbiota or exposure to pathogens (Pabst 2012). Exposure of newborns to microbiota and its subsequent intestinal colonization leads to a progressive increase in the diversity of IgA repertoire (Figure 3). This is due to introduction by microbiota, of mutations in highly expanded B-cell clones and the generation of new mutated B-cell clones (Lindner et al., 2012). Interestingly, the microbiota may also induce mutations in plasma cells to increase diversity of the subsequently produced IgA (Hapfelmeier et al., 2010).

In addition to affecting development and diversity of the immune system, the microbiota induces responses to the intestinal environment that are either for tolerance against most enteral antigens (intestinal microbiota, food antigens and self antigens) or for mounting immune response to eliminate noxious agents that would otherwise bring deleterious effect to the intestinal epithelium. For instance, enteral antigens activate LP plasma cells to produce intestinal IgA that facilitates bacterial translocation through M cells of PP and ILF. This process sensitizes DCs to sample antigens and decide to tolerate or to mount an immune response to non-self or danger signals. The choice depends on the type and amplitude of the microbial challenge as well as intestinal conditioning of the DCs via micro-environmental signals such as retinoic acid and TGF-β (Rey et al., 2004; Coombes and Powrie 2008; Rescigno 2009; Wang et al., 2009).

The microbiota can induce gut tolerance for their antigens. They do this by associating with SIgA in the intestine to enable their entry into the PP via M cells. Subsequently, they are restrictively targeted to tolerogenic DCs for subsequent tolerance (Rol et al., 2012).

It has further been indicated that intestinal dysbacteriosis induced by ceftriaxone in mice reduces immune tolerance in PP and orients the immune response towards humoral immunity by increasing the proportion of $CD4^+/CD8^+$ (Gao et al., 2012).

B Cells and the Microbiota

The production of B cells is partly regulated by microbiota via Treg cells. A study by Cong and others (2009) indicated that depletion of $CD4^{+}CD25^{+}$ Tregs due to microbiotal deficiency decreases IgA^{+} B cells, total IgA, and CBir1-specific IgA in the gut within days. However, repletion of T cell deficient mice with microbiotal-primed $CD4^{+}CD25^{+}$ or $CD4^{+}Foxp3^{+}$ Tregs restores intestinal IgA to a much greater extent than their reciprocal $CD4^{+}$ subsets, indicating that Tregs are the major helper cells for IgA responses to microbiota antigens such as flagellin. Further, production of B cells can be determined by the microbiota since depletion of the commensals impairs production of the B cells. Besides completely depleting gut commensal bacteria, antibiotic treatment diminishes the size of secondary lymphoid tissues such as the PP and decreases the number of B cells and the deposition of both complement 3 and IgM (Yoshiya et al., 2011). This is strong evidence that the microbiota drives the functioning of humoral immunity.

The fact that intestinal microbiotal colonization pattern early in infancy affects the B cell maturation has been demonstrated in experiments involving *Escherichia coli* and *Bifidobacteria*. An early colonization of the gut with these commensals is associated with high numbers of $CD20^{+}$ B cells that express the memory marker CD27 at 4 and 18 months of age (Lundell et al., 2012). Further, the proportion of gut-homing IgG^{+} and IgA^{+} B cells is significantly higher in infants compared with adults. This observation is accounted for by activation of naïve B cells in the gut by microbiota. In fact, it coincides with the establishment of the gut microbiota, suggesting a pivotal role of gut microbiota to the development and establishment of intestinal B cell mediated immunity (Lundell et al., 2011).

IgA and the Microbiota

Contrary to systemic adaptive immunity that is geared at eliminating non-self-antigens, the gut immune system does not eliminate but coexists with gut microbiota and prevents the establishment of harmful bacteria while retaining beneficial and diversified bacteria. To meet this role, the gut immune system produces large amounts of IgA, mainly as dimers or larger polymers, in response to the interaction with gut microbiota. Within the gut lumen, IgA interacts with enteral antigens from the microbiota and food as well as self antigens to control the intestinal microbiota and limit access of these antigens into the bloodstream (Pabst 2012). Most of the IgA responses are generated in the GALT. The dynamic diversification and constant adaptation of IgA responses to local microbiota require expression of AID by B cells and control from T follicular helper (TFH) and Foxp3$^+$ T cells in germinal centers (Figure 4). In addition, Foxp3$^+$ T cells with IgA helper properties, through secretion of TGF-β1, contribute markedly to IgA generation (Nakamura et al., 2001; Tsuji et al., 2009). Th17 cells in PP can also differentiate into TFH cells to support IgA production in the gut (Hirota et al., 2013). Thus there is a clear connection between Foxp3$^+$ T cells, PP germinal centers, IgA, and microbiota in the gut. Disruption of one of these components may have a dramatic impact to the gut immunity. No wonder depletion of Foxp3$^+$ T cells has been shown to cause a rapid loss of microbiotal IgA responses in the gut (Cong et al., 2009; Maynard et al., 2012).

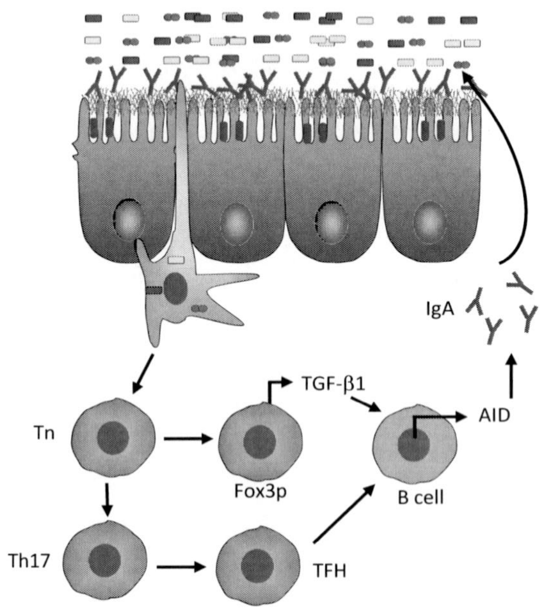

Figure 4. Microbiota-IgA interaction. In a balanced microbiota, dendritic cells sample and present microbiotal antigens to T naïve (Tn) cells and drive differentiation of T helper (Th)17 and Fox3p$^+$ cells. These cells induce expression of AID (activation-induced cytidine deaminase) by B cells to prime production of immunoglobulin (Ig)A. The produced IgA is secreted to the intestinal lumen where it regulates microbiotal profile to maintain intestinal immunity. TFH, T follicular helper; TGF, transforming growth factor.

The LP is the main mucosal effector site where many of IgA-producing cells generated in the PPs relocate and reside. Under normal conditions, the majority of IgAs are induced with the help of $CD4^+$ TFH cells residing in PPs. For preferential switching of B cells in PP germinal centers to IgA, the gut microbiotal and food antigens prime follicular DCs and facilitate activation of TGF-β1 and secretion of B-cell activating factor (BAFF). While TGF-β1 directs switching toward IgA, BAFF maintains survival of recently switched IgA^+ B cells (Suzuki et al., 2010; Cazac and Roes 2000; Mackay and Browning 2002).

The PPs in which the adaptive immune processes take place are already present at birth, since they develop independently of the gut microbiota. However, the formation of germinal centers follows colonization with microbiota. It is in these germinal centers where B cells are activated by microbiotal antigens to express AID and consequently interact with the TFH and $Foxp3^+$ T cells to generate IgA with diversified and adapted responses to local microbiota (Victoria and Nussenzweig 2012; Kato et al., 2013; Ramiscal and Vinuesa 2013). The significance of microbiota to induce formation of germinal centers in PP is explained by the observations that germ-free mice have few if any germinal centers (Cebra et al., 1998; Fagarasan et al., 2010) and that the spontaneous PP germinal center formation and the size of PPs drastically decrease after reduction and/or elimination of gut bacteria by antibiotics (Casola et al., 2004; Zaheen et al., 2009).

The microbiotal induced expression of AID enzyme is vital for B-cell maturation after antigen stimulation. This enzyme triggers class switch recombination (CSR) and somatic hypermutation (SH) of the Ig heavy chain. While CSR modification produces antibodies with different effector functions by switching the B cell receptor class from IgM to IgA, SH introduces non-templated point mutations in the Ig variable region genes, leading to incremented antigen receptor diversity and affinity (Muramatsu et al., 2000; Nagaoka et al., 2010). Within the germinal centers, B cells compete for TFH cell help so that highly mutated B cells with higher affinity to the antigen are generated over their low-mutated counterparts.

For the formation and maintenance of germinal centers and for the generation of most memory B cells and plasma cells, the TFH cells express CD40L, inducible co-stimulator, programmed cell death-1 (PD-1) and OX40 as co-stimulatory molecules and produce IL-21 and IL-4 associated with regulatory and B helper function (Haynes et al., 2007; Crotty 2011; Ramiscal and Vinuesa 2013). The PD-1 is an inhibitory receptor highly expressed on the surface of activated TFH and some B cells. It plays role in shutting down ineffective immune responses and maintaining immune tolerance. Its deficiency causes development of species-specific and antibody-mediated autoimmune disease (Nishimura et al., 1998; Okazaki and Honjo 2006). Mice deficient in PD-1 have a broken immunity exemplified by marked reduction in the number of beneficial *Bifidobacterium*, increased number of more deleterious *Enterobacteriaceae*, hyperplasia of B and T cells, and presence of serum IgG against components of the microbiota. The deregulation of the T cell compartment impacts the selection of IgA plasma cells leading to gut dysbiosis (Kawamoto et al., 2012; Maruya et al., 2013).

Studies have further shown that the microbiota can interact with SIgA to deliver additional tolerogenic signals to antigen sampling DCs to orchestrate non-inflammatory immune responses in the gut (Corthesy 2013). This could be due to the ability of SIgA to interact with receptors of the C-type lectin family that confer tolerogenic properties to DCs such as DC-specific ICAM-3-grabbing non-integrin (DC-SIGN), specific ICAM-3-grabbing non-integrin receptor-1 (SIGNR1), and Dectin-1 (Gutzeit et al., 2014).

It is worth noting that SIgA can limit immune responses against microbiota to contribute to intestinal immune homeostasis (Peterson et al., 2007)

IgA and Microbiota Cross-Talk and Implication during Disease

There is a strong IgA-microbiota cross-talk pertinent to humoral intestinal immunity that plays role during disease. In fact, a balanced indigenous microbiota is required to drive the normal development and functions of mucosal associated lymphoid tissue (MALT), the epithelial barrier, and secretory IgA and IgM system for intestinal immunity. On the contrary, disrupted microbiota predisposes animals to disorders like autoimmunity (Nishimura et al., 1998; Okazaki and Honjo 2006).

The effect of dysbiosis to the intestinal IgA production has been described. Administration of broad spectrum antibiotics that disrupts the commensal microbiota by diminishing up to 2.5-folds the total bacterial counts results in increased luminal SIgA levels and enhanced bacterial wall adhesion (Aguilera et al., 2013). Significantly, these changes impair the gut immunity and predisposes to diseases. It has further been shown in mice that at steady state, the microbiota inhibits transport of both commensal and pathogenic bacteria from the lumen to the MLN, a key immune inductive site. However, in the absence of Myd88 or under conditions of antibiotic-induced dysbiosis, non-invasive bacteria are trafficked to the MLNs in a CCR7-dependent manner, and induce both T-cell responses and IgA production (Diehl et al., 2013).

Deficiency of IgA leads to deregulated microbiotal communities manifested by abnormal expansion of uncultured anaerobes such as segmented filmentous bacteria (SFB) and few species of *Firmicutes* that result in hypersensitivity reactions (Fagarasan et al., 2002; Suzuki et al., 2004). Mice deficient for pIgR, a receptor responsible for epithelial export of IgA and IgM, lack secretory IgA and IgM antibodies and show a variety of defects in their mucosal defense and changes in their intestinal microbiota. Such mice have a reduced epithelial barrier function and increased uptake of antigens from food and commensal bacteria resulting in a hyper-reactive immune system and show predisposition for systemic anaphylaxis after sensitization (Brandtzaeg 2013). A study by Cao and others (2012) reported that commensal antigens trigger Th17 to increase intestinal pIgR and IgA in T cell-deficient TCR-$\beta x \delta^{-/-}$ cells whose pIgR and IgA production is impaired. By regulating the intestinal pIgR expression and IgA secretion the microbiota may potentially overcome impending diseases. Another study by Reikvam and others (2012) consistently found that colonic epithelial cells from pIgR knock-out mice differentially expressed more than 200 genes compared with cells from wild-type mice and upregulated the expression of antimicrobial peptides in a commensal-dependent manner. Detailed profiling of microbial communities revealed differences in the commensal microbiota between pIgR knock-out and wild-type mice. They clearly showed how the absence of pIgR and its subsequent impaired production of IgA and IgM, destabilize the commensal microbiota, compromise the gut homeostasis and worsen the outcome of colitis.

Apart from IgA deficiency, the quality of IgA is crucial for controlling gut microbiota and homeostasis. This is exemplified by an abnormal expansion of *Proteobacteria* and skewed bacterial composition toward *Firmicutes* over *Bacteroidetes* in mice expressing a mutant form of AID (AIDG23S) (Wei et al., 2011).

CONCLUSION

The involvement of microbiota to intestinal humoral immunity is one of interesting gut immune research areas. There is still much to uncover on how the microbiota shapes humoral immune response for gut immunity. Future research focusing on microbiotal role in modulating humoral immune system and protecting the gut could provide more insight into the potential of microbiota in treating several intestinal disorders. Data from such research could be a prelude to designing and producing effective therapeutics against humoral driven intestinal disorders. The potential of microbiota to influence humoral immune responses in health and disease as described herein can be extended to designing medicaments that will improve the host-microbiota interaction and foster intestinal immunity. Current technology employing genomics and designer probiotics could be employed to add potency to microbiota on maintaining intestinal immunity during health and disease.

References

Aguilera, M; Vergara, P; Martínez, V. Stress and antibiotics alter luminal and wall-adhered microbiota and enhance the local expression of visceral sensory-related systems in mice. *Neurogastroenterol Motil.*, 2013, 25, e515-29.

Bouskra, D; Brézillon, C; Bérard, M; et al. Lymphoid tissue genesis induced by commensals through NOD1 regulates intestinal homeostasis. *Nature.*, 2008, 456, 507-510.

Brandtzaeg, P. Secretory IgA: Designed for Anti-Microbial Defense. *Front Immunol.*, 2013, 4, 222.

Brezinschek, HP; Foster, SJ; Brezinschek, RI; et al. Analysis of the human VH gene repertoire. Differential effects of selection and somatic hypermutation on human peripheral CD5(+)/IgM+ and CD5(-)/IgM+ B cells. *J Clin Invest.*, 1997, 99, 2488-2501.

Cao, AT; Yao, S; Gong, B; et al. Th17 cells upregulate polymeric Ig receptor and intestinal IgA and contribute to intestinal homeostasis. *J Immunol.*, 2012, 189, 4666-4673.

Carvalho, FA; Aitken, JD; Vijay-Kumar, M; et al. Toll-like receptor-gut microbiota interactions: perturb at your own risk! *Annu Rev Physiol.*, 2012, 74, 177-198.

Casola, S; Otipoby, KL; Alimzhanov, M; et al. B cell receptor signal strength determines B cell fate. *Nat Immunol.*, 2004, 5, 317-327.

Cazac, BB; Roes, J. TGF-beta receptor controls B cell responsiveness and induction of IgA in vivo. *Immunity.*, 2000, 13, 443-451.

Cebra, JJ; Periwal, SB; Lee, G; et al. Development and maintenance of the gut-associated lymphoid tissue (GALT): the roles of enteric bacteria and viruses. *Dev Immunol.*, 1998, 6, 13-18.

Clarke, TB; Davis, KM; Lysenko, ES; et al. Recognition of peptidoglycan from the microbiota by Nod1 enhances systemic innate immunity. *Nat Med.*, 2010, 16, 228-231.

Cong, Y; Feng, T; Fujihashi, K; et al. A dominant, coordinated T regulatory cell-IgA response to the intestinal microbiota. *Proc Natl Acad Sci USA*, 2009, 106, 19256–19261.

Coombes, JL; Powrie, F. Dendritic cells in intestinal immune regulation. *Nat Rev Immunol.*, 2008, 8, 435-446.

Corthésy, B. Role of secretory IgA in infection and maintenance of homeostasis. *Autoimmun Rev.*, 2013, 12, 661-665.

Crotty, S. Follicular helper CD4 T cells (TFH). *Annu Rev Immunol*, 2011, 29, 621–663.

Cummings, JH; Bingham, SA; Heaton, KW; et al. Fecal weight, colon cancer risk and dietary intake of non-starch polysaccharides (dietary fiber). *Gastroenterology*, 1992, 103, 1408–1412.

Diehl, GE; Longman, RS; Zhang, JX; et al. Microbiota restricts trafficking of bacteria to mesenteric lymph nodes by CX(3)CR1(hi) cells. *Nature.*, 2013, 494, 116-120.

Fagarasan, S; Kawamoto, S; Kanagawa, O; et al. Adaptive immune regulation in the gut: T cell-dependent and T cell-independent IgA synthesis. *Annu Rev Immunol* 2010, 28, 243–273.

Fagarasan, S; Kinoshita, K; Muramatsu, M; et al. In situ class switching and differentiation to IgA-producing cells in the gut lamina propria. *Nature.*, 2001, 413, 639-643.

Fagarasan, S; Muramatsu, M; Suzuki, K; et al. Critical roles of activation-induced cytidine deaminase in the homeostasis of gut flora. *Science.*, 2002, 298, 1424-1427.

Gao, F; Li, M; Liu, Y; et al. Intestinal dysbacteriosis induces changes of T lymphocyte subpopulations in Peyer's patches of mice and orients the immune response towards humoral immunity. *Gut Pathog.*, 2012, 4, 19.

Garrett, WS; Gallini, CA; Yatsunenko, T; et al. Enterobacteriaceae act in concert with the gut microbiota to induce spontaneous and maternally transmitted colitis. *Cell Host Microbe.*, 2010, 8, 292-300.

Gutzeit, C; Magri, G; Cerutti, A. Intestinal IgA production and its role in host-microbe interaction. *Immunol Rev.*, 2014, 260, 76-85.

Hannet, I; Erkeller-Yuksel, F; Lydyard, P; et al. Developmental and maturational changes in human blood lymphocyte subpopulations. *Immunol Today.*, 1992, 13, 215, 218.

Hapfelmeier, S; Lawson, MA; Slack, E; et al. Reversible microbial colonization of germ-free mice reveals the dynamics of IgA immune responses. *Science.*, 2010, 328, 1705-1709.

Haynes, NM; Allen, CD; Lesley, R; et al. Role of CXCR5 and CCR7 in follicular Th cell positioning and appearance of a programmed cell death gene-1high germinal center-associated subpopulation. *J Immunol.*, 2007, 179, 5099-5108.

He, B; Xu, W; Santini, PA; et al. Intestinal bacteria trigger T cell-independent immunoglobulin A(2) class switching by inducing epithelial-cell secretion of the cytokine APRIL. *Immunity.*, 2007, 26, 812-826.

Hirota, K; Turner, JE; Villa, M; et al. Plasticity of Th17 cells in Peyer's patches is responsible for the induction of T cell-dependent IgA responses. *Nat Immunol*, 2013, 14, 372–379.

Hugot, JP; Chamaillard, M; Zouali, H; et al. Association of NOD2 leucine-rich repeat variants with susceptibility to Crohn's disease. *Nature.*, 2001, 411(6837), 599-603.

Imaoka, A; Matsumoto, S; Setoyama, H; et al. Proliferative recruitment of intestinal intraepithelial lymphocytes after microbial colonization of germ-free mice. *Eur J Immunol.*, 1996, 26, 945-948.

Izcue, A; Coombes, JL; Powrie, F. Regulatory lymphocytes and intestinal inflammation. *Annu Rev Immunol.*, 2009, 27, 313-38.

Johansson, ME; Sjovall, H; Hansson, GC. The gastrointestinal mucus system in health and disease. *Nat Rev Gastroenterol Hepatol*, 2013, 10, 352–361.

Johansson-Lindbom, B; Agace, WW. Generation of gut-homing T cells and their localization to the small intestinal mucosa. *Immunol Rev.*, 2007, 215, 226-242.

Kato, LM; Kawamoto, S; Maruya, M; et al. Gut TFH and IgA: key players for regulation of bacterial communities and immune homeostasis. *Immunol Cell Biol.*, 2014, 92, 49-56.

Kawamoto, S; Tran, TH; Maruya, M; et al. The inhibitory receptor PD-1 regulates IgA selection and bacterial composition in the gut. *Science.*, 2012, 336, 485-489.

Kunkel, D; Kirchhoff, D; Nishikawa, S; et al. Visualization of peptide presentation following oral application of antigen in normal and Peyer's patches-deficient mice. *Eur J Immunol.*, 2003, 33, 1292-1301.

Lindner, C; Wahl, B; Föhse, L; et al. Age, microbiota, and T cells shape diverse individual IgA repertoires in the intestine. *J Exp Med.*, 2012, 209, 365-377.

Locke, NR; Stankovic, S; Funda, DP; et al. TCR gamma delta intraepithelial lymphocytes are required for self-tolerance. *J Immunol.*, 2006, 176, 6553-6559.

Lundell, AC; Björnsson, V; Ljung, A; et al. Infant B cell memory differentiation and early gut bacterial colonization. *J Immunol.*, 2012, 188, 4315-4322.

Lundell, AC; Rabe, H; Quiding-Järbrink, M; et al. Development of gut-homing receptors on circulating B cells during infancy. *Clin Immunol.*, 2011, 138, 97-106.

Mackenzie, LE; Youinou, PY; Hicks, R; et al. Auto- and polyreactivity of IgM from CD5+ and CD5- cord blood B cells. *Scand J Immunol.*, 1991, 33, 329-335.

Maruya, M; Kawamoto, S; Kato, LM; et al. Impaired selection of IgA and intestinal dysbiosis associated with PD-1-deficiency. *Gut Microbes.*, 2013, 4, 165-171.

Maynard, CL; Elson, CO; Hatton, RD; et al. Reciprocal interactions of the intestinal microbiota and immune system. *Nature.*, 2012, 489, 231–241.

Mestecky, J; McGhee, JR. Immunoglobulin A (IgA): molecular and cellular interactions involved in IgA biosynthesis and immune response. *Adv Immunol.*, 1987, 40, 153–245.

Mora, JR; von, Andrian, UH. Role of retinoic acid in the imprinting of gut-homing IgA-secreting cells. *Semin Immunol.*, 2009, 21, 28–35.

Muramatsu, M; Kinoshita, K; Fagarasan, S; et al. Class switch recombination and hypermutation require activation-induced cytidine deaminase (AID), a potential RNA editing enzyme. *Cell.*, 2000, 102, 553-563.

Nagaoka, H; Tran, TH; Kobayashi, M; et al. Preventing AID, a physiological mutator, from deleterious activation: regulation of the genomic instability that is associated with antibody diversity. *Int Immunol.*, 2010, 22, 227-235.

Nakamura, K; Kitani, A; Strober, W. Cell contact-dependent immunosuppression by CD4(þ)CD25(þ) regulatory T cells is mediated by cell surface-bound transforming growth factor beta. *J Exp Med*, 2001, 194, 629–644.

Nishimura, H; Minato, N; Nakano, T; et al. Immunological studies on PD-1 deficient mice: implication of PD-1 as a negative regulator for B cell responses. *Int Immunol*, 1998, 10, 1563–1572.

Okazaki, T; Honjo, T. The PD-1-PD-L pathway in immunological tolerance. *Trends Immunol.*, 2006, 27, 195-201.

Pabst, O. New concepts in the generation and functions of IgA. *Nat Rev Immunol.*, 2012, 12, 821–832.

Peterson, DA; McNulty, NP; Guruge, JL; et al. IgA response to symbiotic bacteria as a mediator of gut homeostasis. *Cell Host Microbe.*, 2007, 2, 328-339.

Phalipon, A; Cardona, A; Kraehenbuhl, JP; et al. Secretory component: a new role in secretory IgA-mediated immune exclusion in vivo. *Immunity.*, 2002, 17, 107–115.

Ramiscal, RR; Vinuesa, CG. T-cell subsets in the germinal center. *Immunol Rev.*, 2013, 252, 146–155.

Reikvam, DH; Derrien, M; Islam, R; et al. Epithelial-microbial crosstalk in polymeric Ig receptor deficient mice. *Eur J Immunol.*, 2012, 42, 2959-2970.

Rescigno, M. Before they were gut dendritic cells. *Immunity.*, 2009, 31, 454-456.

Rescigno, M. Functional specialization of antigen presenting cells in the gastrointestinal tract. *Curr Opin Immunol.*, 2010, 22, 131-136.

Rescigno, M. Intestinal dendritic cells. *Adv Immunol.*, 2010, 107, 109-138.

Rey J, Garin N, Spertini F, et al. Targeting of secretory IgA to Peyer's patch dendritic and T cells after transport by intestinal M cells. *J Immunol.*, 2004, 172, 3026-3033.

Rol, N; Favre, L; Benyacoub, J; et al. The role of secretory immunoglobulin A in the natural sensing of commensal bacteria by mouse Peyer's patch dendritic cells. *J Biol Chem.*, 2012, 287, 40074-40082

Salminen, S; Bouley, C; Boutron-Ruault, MC; et al. Functional food science and gastrointestinal physiology and function. *Br J Nutr.*, 1998, 80 Suppl 1, S147-171.

Schenk, M; Mueller, C. The mucosal immune system at the gastrointestinal barrier. *Best Pract Res Clin Gastroenterol.*, 2008, 22, 391-409.

Sekirov, I; Russell, SL; Antunes, LC; et al. Gut microbiota in health and disease. *Physiol Rev.*, 2010, 90, 859-904.

Stall, AM; Wells, SM; Lam, KP. B-1 cells: unique origins and functions. *Semin Immunol.*, 1996, 8, 45-59.

Strowig, T; Henao-Mejia, J; Elinav, E; et al. Inflammasomes in health and disease. *Nature.*, 2012, 481, 278-286.

Strugnell, RA; Wijburg, OL. The role of secretory antibodies in infection *immunity. Nat Rev Microbiol*, 2010, 8, 656–667.

Suzuki, K; Maruya, M; Kawamoto, S; et al. The sensing of environmental stimuli by follicular dendritic cells promotes immunoglobulin A generation in the gut. *Immunity.*, 2010, 33, 71-83.

Suzuki, K; Meek, B; Doi, Y; et al. Two distinctive pathways for recruitment of naive and primed IgM+ B cells to the gut lamina propria. *Proc Natl Acad Sci U S A.*, 2005, 102, 2482-2486.

Suzuki, K; Meek, B; Doi, Y; et al. Aberrant expansion of segmented filamentous bacteria in IgA-deficient gut. *Proc Natl Acad Sci U S A.*, 2004, 101, 1981-1986.

Tap, J; Mondot, S; Levenez, F; et al. Towards the human intestinal microbiota phylogenetic core. *Environ Microbiol.*, 2009, 11, 2574-2584.

Tsuji, M; Komatsu, N; Kawamoto, S; et al. Preferential generation of follicular B helper T cells from Foxp3þ T cells in gut Peyer's patches. *Science*, 2009, 323, 1488–1492.

Vaishnava, S; Behrendt, CL; Ismail, AS; et al. Paneth cells directly sense gut commensals and maintain homeostasis at the intestinal host-microbial interface. *Proc Natl Acad Sci U S A.*, 2008, 105, 20858-20863.

Victora, GD; Nussenzweig, MC. Germinal centers. *Annu Rev Immunol.*, 2012, 30, 429-457.

Voss, RH; Kuball, J; Engel, R; et al. Redirection of T cells by delivering a transgenic mouse-derived MDM2 tumor antigen-specific TCR and its humanized derivative is governed by the CD8 coreceptor and affects natural human TCR expression. *Immunol Res.*, 2006, 34, 67-87.

Wang, J; Huizinga, TW; Toes, RE. De novo generation and enhanced suppression of human CD4+CD25+ regulatory T cells by retinoic acid. *J Immunol.*, 2009, 183, 4119-4126.

Wei, M; Shinkura, R; Doi, Y; et al. Mice carrying a knock-in mutation of Aicda resulting in a defect in somatic hypermutation have impaired gut homeostasis and compromised mucosal defense. *Nat Immunol.*, 2011, 12, 264-270.

Williams, AM; Probert, CS; Stepankova, R; et al. Effects of microflora on the neonatal development of gut mucosal T cells and myeloid cells in the mouse. *Immunology.*, 2006, 119, 470-478.

Xavier, RJ; Podolsky, DK. Unravelling the pathogenesis of inflammatory bowel disease. *Nature.*, 2007, 448, 427-434.

Yoshiya, K; Lapchak, PH; Thai, TH; et al. Depletion of gut commensal bacteria attenuates intestinal ischemia/reperfusion injury. *Am J Physiol Gastrointest Liver Physiol.*, 2011, 301, G1020-G1030.

Zaheen, A; Boulianne, B; Parsa, JY; et al. AID constrains germinal center size by rendering B cells susceptible to apoptosis. *Blood.*, 2009, 114, 547-554.

Chapter 5

MICROBIOTAL INFLUENCE ON T CELL FUNCTIONING DURING INTESTINAL HEALTH AND DISEASE

ABSTRACT

T cell response forms the cellular part of intestinal adaptive immune system. The response is usually elicited following encounter of T cells with antigens presented by antigen presentating cells like macrophages, dendritic cells or B cells. Competent immune cells in this system include T helper, regulatory T, cytotoxic T, memory T, natural killer T, and mucosa associated invariant T cells. Most, if not all, of these cells produce mediators that drive pro- or anti-inflammatory, cytotoxic, and proliferative functions during health and disease depending upon the stimulating antigens. Antigens from balanced intestinal microbiota drive tolerogenic responses whereas those from pathogens and disrupted microbiota induce immune responses that cause inflammation and disease. In some instances, maneuvers that restore to normal the disrupted microbiota during disease, benefits patients by reducing or ameliorating the severity of the disease. The significance of microbiota to T cell responses and their subsequent effect on individual's health stems, at least in part, from the large number and diverse microbiotal antigens found in intestinal lumen. Understanding the influence of this diverse microbiota to T cell responses during health and disease is the intention of this chapter.

Introduction

The vast injurious agents including extrinsic pathogens and their products, xenobiotics, chemicals, thermal and related stress stimuli and intrinsic genetic aberrations, cancer cells, and inflammatory cytokines together with food proteins and highly diverse microbiota are exposed to the gut immune system at any time in an individual's lifetime. Such an exposure triggers both innate and acquired immune systems to respond in a way that discriminates between injurious and non-harmful food proteins and microbiota. Similar to other body systems, the gut acquired immune system comprises cellular and humoral components. The cellular component is predominated by T cells whose population is highest in the gastrointestinal tract than other body systems. This can be attributed to the constant exposure of the gut to the diverse antigens emanating from extrinsic and intrinsic agents. The diverse gut antigenic environment has made T cells to be highly plastic and readily capable of differentiating into new phenotypes with respect to antigenic stimuli (Feng et al., 2011). T cells are therefore heterogeneous in their membrane receptors as well as effector responses. They are regulated by several factors including microbiota and pathogens via their microbe-associated molecular patterns (MAMPs), microbial and host metabolites, hormones, and inflammatory mediators such as cytokines. Among these factors, cytokines are the most encountered and potent triggers of T cell activation, expansion, differentiation, and survival. While retinoic acid plays critical role in regulating T cell differentiation, migration, and effector responses in the small intestine, the large number and diversity of microbes in the colon are sufficient to carry out similar role in the large intestine (Kim 2013).

The main components of T cells that sustain the cellular acquired immune system are $CD4^+$ cells which include T helper (Th) and regulatory T (Treg) cells (Mosmann and Coffman 1989; Atarashi et al., 2011; Feng and Elson 2011; Kim et al., 2013). Other T cells like cytotoxic (Tc), memory, natural killer (NKT), and mucosa associated invariant T cells may also contribute to intestinal immunity to variable degrees (Tanaka et al., 2007; Hand et al., 2012; Zeissig and Blumberg 2013; Olszak et al., 2014). However, the specific roles of most of these cells to the gut immunity are not fully established although they converge at maintaining immune homeostasis through imparting tolerance or inciting active immune responses. While T cell reactions against endogenous antigens may lead to autoimmune diseases, failure or excessive reaction of the T cell response to non-self antigens leads to immune disorders that could either be immunodeficiency or hypersensitivity, respectively.

Furthermore, challenges to the gut by these agents may lead to breakdown of the immune system and subsequent development of non-immune mediated gastrointestinal diseases.

The influence of microbiota to the gut immunity is enormous. Its overwhelming number (about 10 times the total body cells of an individual) and wide antigenic diversity (6-10 phyla and approximately up to 5,000 distinct species of bacteria) (Tap et al., 2009; Garrett et al., 2010; Carvalho et al., 2012), allude to its essential role to gut immunity. It drives T cells to generate responses designated at discriminating antigens from non harmful microbiota and deleterious invaders to maintain immune homeostasis. In particular, to modulate T cell functions, the microbiota influences growth of T cells (Wei et al., 2010; Wingender et al., 2012; Mittrücker et al., 2014), differentiation (Wei et al., 2010; Hand et al., 2012; Wingender et al., 2012) antigen presentation, production of inflammatory cytokines (Bouma and Strober 2003; Weaver et al., 2013), and polarization of T-cell driven responses (Bouma and Strober 2003). These functions are so essential to the gut immunity that absence of microbiota (e.g., germ-free animals) and/or disruption in the balance of microbiota profile, lead to T-cell mediated disorders like inflammatory bowel disease (IBD), several types of colitides, irritable bowel syndrome (IBS), and allergy (Sekirov et al., 2010). For instance, the microbiota-dependent T-cell homing into the intestinal lamina propria (LP) to cause tolerance is lost during deficiency of microbiota leading to serious inflammation (Kim et al., 2013). Thus, although T cells drive gut immunity, on the dark side they are pivotal to development of gut immune mediated diseases, especially following disruption or deficiency of microflora. Most of such diseases affect the large bowel which has higher number (up to 1×10^{12} bacterial cells per gram of colonic content) and diversity of microbiota (McGuckin et al., 2011) and more frequencies of T cells (Atarashi et al., 2011; Geuking et al., 2011) than the small intestine. These facts suggest that the microbiota plays a vital role in sustaining the gut immunity, especially in locations where they are normally high in number and diversity. In this chapter the influence of microbiota to the functioning of intestinal T cells during health and disease is described.

T CELLS

T cells or T lymphocytes include Th, Treg, Tc, NKT, memory, and mucosa associated invariant T cells. Th cells express CD4 molecules on their surface and are thus called $CD4^+$ T cells. They recognize antigens presented in association with major histocompatibility class (MHC)II expressed by antigen presenting cells (APCs) and respond by rapid proliferation and production of various cytokines including interleukin (IL)-1β, IL-2, IL-4, IL5, IL-6, IL-8, IL-10, IL-12, IL-17, IL-22, and IL-23 (Evrard et al., 2011; Feng and Elson 2011; Schiavi et al., 2011; Weaver et al., 2013). The $CD4^+$ T cells drive the differentiation of B cells into plasma and memory cells and activate Tc cells and macrophages. They include Th1, Th2, Th3, Th9, Th17 and follicular helper T (TFH) cells. Treg cells were formerly called suppressor T cells. They are essential for maintaining intestinal immune tolerance by suppressing T cell responses after immune reaction as well as auto-reactive T cells. NKT cells link innate and adaptive immune systems. They recognize self- and microbial glycolipids presented by CD1d molecule instead of MHC as is the case with other T cells and respond by producing cytokines and cytolytic chemicals. They also eliminate viral infected and tumor cells. The role of Tc cells is to eliminate viral infected and tumor cells, reject grafts and prevent autoimmune diseases. They express CD8 molecules and recognize antigens associated with MHCI molecules. They are involved in many autoimmune diseases. Memory T cells are antigen-specific cells originating from T cells previously exposed to an antigen. Upon encounter to the same antigen, they proliferate to large numbers of effector T cells to protect against the particular antigen. They are either $CD4^+$ or $CD8^+$ and include central memory T (Tcm) and effector memory T (Tem and Temra) cells (Willinger et al., 2005).

EFFECTOR T CELLS

Effector T cells shown to play a role in the gut immunity to encounter a large number and diverse array of microbiota, commensal fungi, and food antigens include Th1, Th2, Th17, and TFH $CD4^+$ T cells. However, there are few $CD8^+$ and invariant NKT (iNKT) cells located within the germinal centers of intestinal Peyer's patches (PP). The effector T cells play a key role in the regulation of both innate and adaptive immunity. Their classification and identification are based on their products (Th1, Th2, and Th17) or expression of homing receptor (TFH) that eventually define their function.

Th1 cells produce interferon (IFN)-γ, a potent activator of innate immune cells, particularly macrophages. This response fights against intracellular pathogens that evade the microbicidal functions of phagocytes. IFN-γ also promotes class-switch of B cells to immunoglobulin (Ig)G that opsonize microbes for enhanced uptake by phagocytes (Figure 1). Th2 cells produce IL-4, IL-5, and IL-13 (Mosmann and Coffman 1989) to fight against parasitic infections like helminths primarily from mucosal sites of infection. They also coordinate B cell class switching to produce IgE that lead to degranulation of basophils and mast cells (IL-4 and IL-13), enhanced eosinophil mobilization (IL-5), and increased mucus production and hypermotility (IL-13) during allergic reactions (Mosmann and Coffman 1989)

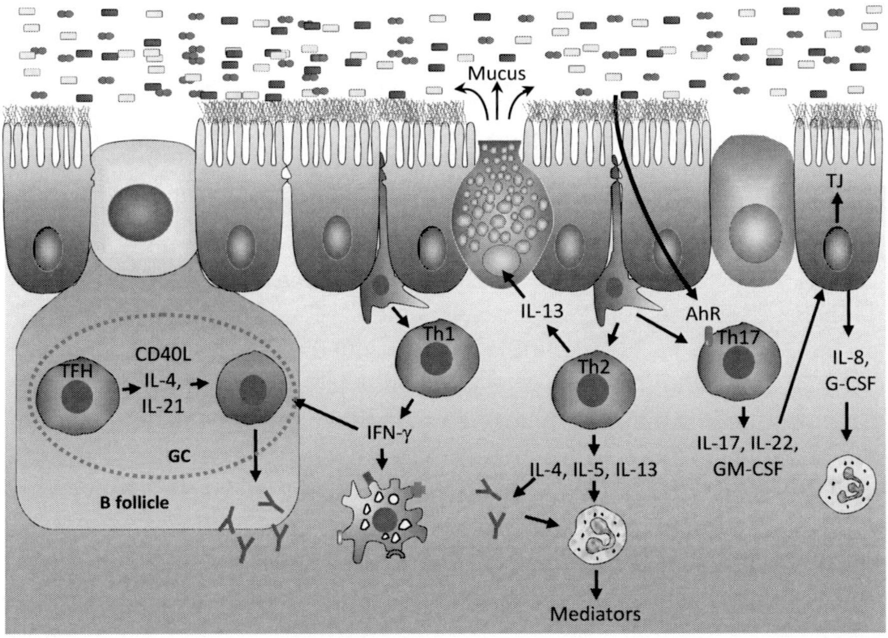

Figure 1. Microbiotal-mediated effector T cell functioning. Dendritic cell sampling and presentation of microbiota antigens to T cells drive the phenotype of Th1, Th2 and Th17 manifested by production of various inflammatory cytokines. The produced cytokines activate B cells, macrophages, eosinophils and neutrophils whose responses maintain intestinal immunity during health and disease. B cell-mediated production of immunoglobulins is further driven by follicular T helper (TFH) in B follicle germinal centers (GC). Ahr, aryl hydrocarbon receptor; G-CSF, granulocyte colony stimulating factor; IFN, interferon; IL, interleukin.

Th17 cells produce IL-17 family cytokines (IL-17A and IL-17F), IL-22 (a member of IL-10), and granulocyte macrophage colony-stimulating factor

(GM-CSF). IL-17 cytokines mainly target innate immune cells and epithelial cells to produce granulocyte colony stimulating factor (G-CSF) and IL-8 (CXCL8), which induce increased neutrophil production and recruitment, respectively. IL-22 acts on epithelial cells of mucosal barrier and the skin to fight against microbes and institute epithelial barrier integrity. GM-CSF promotes enhanced bone marrow production of granulocytes and monocytes (Feng and Elson 2011; Weaver et al., 2013). The Th17 cells share developmental requirements for the transcription factor retinoic acid-related orphan receptor (ROR)γt and the aryl hydrocarbon receptor (Ahr) with intestinal innate lymphoid cells. RORγt is essential for Th17 development and function whereas Ahr is used for sensing microbiota metabolites and xenobiotics (Sawa et al., 2011). Furthermore, Th17 cells have developmental ties with Treg cells through their mutual requirement for the abundant intestinal cytokine transforming growth factor (TGF)-β (Weaver and Hatton 2009). The Th1, Th2 and Th17 effector T cells appear to specialize in augmenting and coordinating the functions of gut adaptive immunity in which case, Th1 works for monocyte/macrophages responses, Th2 cells go for eosinophils, basophils, and mast cells and Th17 cells mainly focus on neutrophils (Figure 1). TFH are $CD4^+$ T cells found in the germinal centers of B cell follicles of PP. They are produced following induction of Bcl6 protein and are identified by their ability to express the B cell follicle homing receptor CXCR5 (Fazilleau 2009). There are two major kinds of these cells; TFH cells, defined as $CXCR5^+PD\text{-}1^{hi}Foxp3^-$ cells, and T follicular regulatory (TFR) cells, defined as $CXCR5^+PD\text{-}1^{hi}Foxp3^+$ cells (Linterman et al., 2011; Chung et al., 2011). TFH cells mediate antigen specific naïve or memory B cell activation to form germinal centers through the expression of CD40L and the secretion of IL-21 and IL-4 (Seo et al., 2009; Zaretsky et al., 2009). Although it is possible that TFH cells might arise as branches in the Th1 and Th2 differentiation pathways, several studies have shown that TFH have distinct gene expression profiles and may thus be a subset of $CD4^+$ T cells distinct from Th1, Th2, Th17 or Tregs (Chtanova et al., 2004; Nurieve et al., 2008).

Influence of Microbiota on Effector T Cells during Health and Disease

A clear link between effector T cells and the gut microbiota is evident right from the development of the T cells to their operation. Hrncir and others

(2008) found that the gut microbiota and to a lesser extent the lipopolysaccharide (LPS)-rich sterile diet drive the expansion of B and T cells in PP and mesenteric lymph nodes (MLN). The most prominent is the expansion of CD4$^+$ T cells including Foxp3$^+$ T cells in MLN (Figure 2). Recently, Jakobsson and others observed that caesarian born children have lower microbiota diversity and delayed colonization by *Bacteroidetes* than vaginally born children in the first two years of life. This predisposes them to reduced Th1 responses (Jakobsson et al., 2014). These studies and several others indicate clearly that live gut microbiota diversity as well as microbial components (LPS) stimulate the development, expansion and function of the gut immune system.

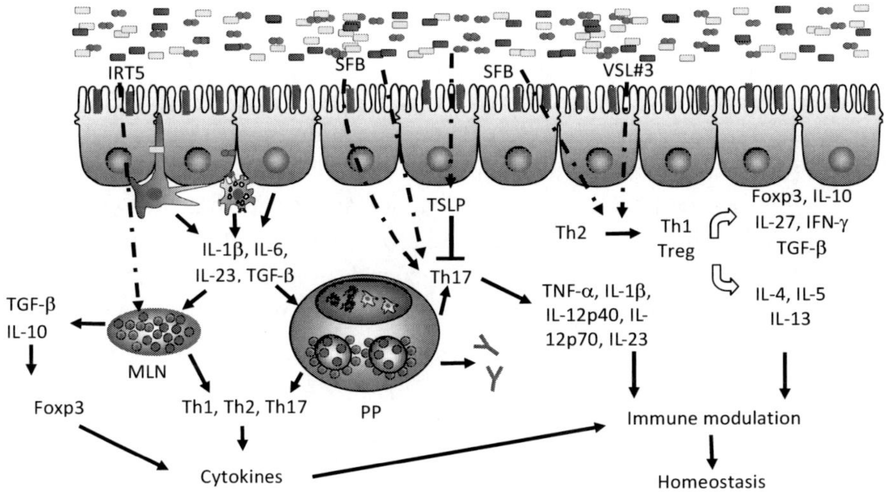

Figure 2. Influence of microbiota on effector T cell responses. The microbiota and specific commensal bacterial species induce expansion of effector T cells (Th1, Th2, Th17) in the Payer's patches (PP) and mesenteric lymph nodes (MLN). The effector Th2 can also switch into Th1 or regulatory T (Treg) cells under the influence of microbiota or specific microbiotal member species. Subsequently, the effector T or Treg cells produce inflammatory cytokines that modulate the immune system to induce homeostasis.

For the development of Th17 cells, the contribution of microbioata is appreciated by the virtual absence of this subset in germ-free mice (Ivanov et al., 2008). This is partly due to lack of microbioata-dependent factors that favour development of Th17. Such factors could include IL-6 required for Th17 differentiation and its deviation away from induced Treg programming,

TGF-β, IL-1β, IL-23, and ATP derived from commensal bacteria (Figure 2) (Maynard et al., 2012). It has recently been established that the microbiota constitutively maintains substantial levels of intestinal thymic stromal lymphopoietin (TSLP) that regulates colitis by limiting the expansion of Th17 cells. Disruption of the microbiota and its subsequent perturbed TSLP activity leads to inappropriate control of Th17 expansion that could predispose to colitis (Mosconi et al., 2013).

Ubiquitous presence of Th17 cells in the intestinal LP at steady state is controlled by microbiota. In this regard, the microbiota triggers macrophages to produce IL-1β which directly drives differentiation of IL-1R-expressing T cells into intestinal steady state Th17 (Shaw et al., 2012). The *Clostridia* sp. *Candidatus arthromitus* or segmented filamentous bacteria (SFB) have been observed to be a potent minor constituent of the microbiota that induces development of Th17 cells (Geuking et al., 2011). This is manifested by an association between the presence or absence of SFB and the number of Th17 cells in the intestinal LP (Figure 2). The association is such that the presence of SFB induces a dramatic increase in Th17 cells (Ivanov et al., 2009; Salzman et al., 2010). Recently, Geem and colleagues suggested that SFB creates an intestinal milieu that drives the differentiation of intestinal $CD4^+$ naïve T into Th17 cells in response to food and/or bacterial antigens (Geem et al., 2014). Further, mono-colonization of mice by SFB promotes the generation of intestinal Th17 cells (together with IgA plasma cells) and enhances the expression of IFN-γ and Foxp3 in gut T cell subsets (Gaboriau-Routhiau et al., 2009). The specific microbiota SFB, has also been shown to modulate the activation threshold of self-reactive T cells in a Th1-cell-driven murine model of autoimmune arthritis. In this model, the commensal flora elicited inflammatory cytokines in the local microenvironment of GALT that dynamically enhanced the antigen responsiveness of T cells that were otherwise tuned down to a systemic self-antigen (Chappert et al., 2013). Intestinal colonization by SFB also primes Th17 cell antigen receptor (TCR) repertoire to specifically focus on SFB antigens and differentiate into RORγt-expressing Th17 cells. These changes occur even in the presence of strong inducers of Th1 cells, indicating that the microbiota can strongly determine the match between T-cell effector function and antigen specificity (Yang et al., 2014).

Another study indicated that oral VSL#3 (composes of *Lactobacillus casei*, *L. plantarum*, *L. acidophilus*, *L. delbrueckii* subsp. *bulgaricus*, *B. longum*, *Bifidobacterium infantis*, *B. breve*, and *Streptococcus salivarius* subsp. *thermophilus*) treatment of mice sensitized to a major food allergen, shrimp tropomyocin, shifted a polarized Th2 response to a Th1/Treg response leading to a decrease in IL-4, IL-5, and IL-13 production and an increase in Foxp3, IL-10, IL-27, IFN-γ, and TGF-β in the jejunum (Figure 2) (Schiavi et al., 2011). Further, administration of IRT5 microbial mixture (contains *L. acidophilus, L. casei, L. reuteri, Bifidobacterium bifidium,* and *Streptococcus thermophilus*), induced high levels of IL-10, TGF-β, and indoleamine 2,3-dioxygenase (IDO) in MLN CD11c$^+$ dendritic cells (DCs), which promoted the generation of Foxp3 Treg cells in inflamed areas of murine models of IBD, atopic dermatitis, and rheumatoid arthritis (Figure 2). Interestingly, DCs isolated from the IRT5-fed mice effectively induced the differentiation of CD4$^+$ T cells into CD4$^+$Foxp3$^+$ iTregs contrary to DCs from control animals (Kwon et al., 2010; Chae et al., 2012).

Orally administered commensal microbes have been shown to modulate the adaptive immune system in a dose dependent manner. Exposure of DCs to high doses of *Lactobacillus rhamnosus* Lcr35 induces a Th1/Th17 skewing cytokine profile manifested by high levels of TNF-α, IL-1β, IL-12p40, IL-12p70, and IL-23 and low levels of IL-10. There is also an increase in the expression of markers of maturity such as CD86, CD83, HLA-DR and TLR4 by DCs. On the contrary, low doses of this commensal do not change the expression of pro- or anti-inflammatory genes and the markers of maturity are indicative of immature DCs (Evrard et al., 2011). The orally administered commensal microbes that can affect the microbiota profile in the gut can thus, have different effects on the immune system depending on the dose and frequency of administration.

Apart from the dose effect, a species- and strain-specific modulation of the immune system by microbiota has been reported. By analyzing the cytokine profile of bone marrow-derived DCs stimulated by 27 different lactobacilli and 16 bifidobacteria, Weiss and others (2011) found that different groups of lactobacilli have distinct and opposite effects on IL-12, TNF-α, and IFN-γ secretion by DCs while all bifidobacteria tested decreased the production these cytokines. They also found that *L. acidophilus* NCFM induces Th1 skewing pro-inflammatory cytokine profile which can be down-regulated by *B. bifidum* Z9 (Weiss et al., 2010). This observation could indicate that commensal bacteria selectively modulate the immune system for gut homeostasis during health or disease. Consistently, Cao and other (2012) demonstrated that the microbiota-specific effector T cells, particularly Th17 cells, contribute to intestinal homeostasis by regulating intestinal polymeric Ig receptor (pIgR) expression and IgA secretion. In so doing, they can protect against intestinal inflammation (Cao et al., 2012). Yet a more recent study by Konieczna and others (2013) observed that *Bifidobacterium infantis* 35624 feeding to mice resulted in increased numbers of $CD103^+$ retinaldehyde dehydrogenase $(RALDH)^+$ DCs within the LP. $Foxp3^+$ lymphocytes were also increased in the LP, while Th1 and Th17 subsets were decreased. In addition, *B. infantis* reduced the severity of dextran sulfate sodium (DSS)-induced colitis, associated with decreased Th1 and Th17 cells within the LP. Indeed, $CD103^+$ $RALDH^+$ LP DCs are important cellular targets for microbiota-associated effects on mucosal immunoregulation that involves the effector Th1 and Th17 cells.

TREG CELLS

Treg cells are a component of the immune system that balances between pro- and anti-inflammatory responses at mucosal surfaces and suppresses immune responses of other cells to prevent excessive reactions. The end result of this regulatory role is induction of tolerance and prevention of immune-mediated disorders for maintenance of gut homeostasis. Imbalanced function or number of these cells may lead to tumor development and autoimmunity.

Treg cells are classified as natural Treg (nTreg) (also called thymic) and inducible Treg (iTreg) (also called peripherally induced) cells. The nTreg cells are the $Foxp3^+CD4^+CD25^+$ T cells developed as a distinct lineage in the thymus. They are the most potent Treg cells accounting for about 10% of peripheral $CD4^+$ T cells. Their main role is to maintain tolerance toward self-structures. To meet this function, they acquire tissue specific features and a diversified pattern of homing receptors as well as becoming adapted to function within the tissues of their residency (Kim et al., 2013).

Inducible Treg cells comprise $CD4^+CD8^+$ T cells generated from peripheral naïve conventional T (Tconv) cells through induction of transcription factor, Foxp3 in response to low immunogenic doses of externally or intestinal delivered antigens, commensal microbes, lymphopenia, activation by immature DCs, co-stimulation from APCs and can be generated *in vitro* (Curotto de Lafaille and Lafaille, 2009; Atarashi et al., 2011). Within intestinal lymphoid compartments iTreg cells receive homing cues, which direct these cells to the gut LP where they expand and locally suppress immune responses to maintain homeostasis. They are subdivided on the basis of their expression of Foxp3 into $Foxp3^+$ (Treg) (e.g., Treg17) and $Foxp3^-$ Treg cells 1 (Tr1), Th3 (a TGF-β-producing Treg), $CD8^+CD28^+$, and Qa-1 restricted T cells. Although the contribution of these populations to self-tolerance and immune homeostasis is less well defined, both iTreg classes induce production of a prominent anti-inflammatory cytokine, IL-10, pivotal to immune tolerance of the intestinal microbiota.

INFLUENCE OF MICROBIOTA ON TREG DURING HEALTH AND DISEASE

Although traditionally thymic and induced Treg cells are known to mediate self and non-self antigens respectively, recent findings indicate that the microbiota heavily influences thymic rather than induced Treg cells to mediate tolerance to microbiota antigens (Cebula et al., 2013). The microbiota also regulates the balance between pro- and anti-inflammatory responses of T cells via its carbohydrate fermentation products, short chain fatty acids (SCFAs). This is achieved through histone deacetylase (HDAC) inhibition by SCFAs which induces generation of Treg cells by potentiating extrathymic differentiation of Treg cells in a conserved non-coding sequence (CNS)1-dependent fashion (Arpaia et al., 2013). Studies have further indicated that first exposure to microbiota in early life is crucial for Treg cell functioning throughout an individual's life. According to Hansen and colleagues, at weaning, caesarean section born mice exhibit higher numbers of *Bacteroides* and *Lachnospiraceae* and less *Rikenellaceae* and *Ruminococcus* than vaginally born mice. However, at adulthood caesarean section born mice have less Foxp3$^+$ Treg cells than vaginally born animals. This variation may have ramification on development of immune mediated disease like diabetes mellitus in adulthood (Hansen et al., 2014).

The influence of microbiota to Treg cells is further depicted in the plasticity of these cells. Intestinal Treg (Foxp3$^+$) cells derived from naïve T cells convert, under the influence of microbiota into IFN-γ^+ Th1, IL-17$^+$ Th17, and Foxp3$^+$ Treg cells coexpressing IFN- and/or IL-17 (Figure 3). In its transition stage, the generated Foxp3$^+$IFN-γ^+ T cells retain their regulatory function and suppress proliferation of naïve T cells to inhibit induction of colitis (Feng et al., 2011). The microbiota-induced proliferation and functional maturity of intestinal Treg cells is mediated by overexpression of DNA-methylation adaptor Uhrf1 in Treg cells. The Uhrf1 activates Cdkn1a gene encoding cyclin-dependent kinase inhibitor p21 responsible for cell-cycle activity. Gut immunological homeostasis is achieved by microbiota-mediated

Uhrf1-dependent silencing of Cdkn1a gene activation whereas deficiency of Uhrf1 predisposes mice to spontaneously severe colitis (Obata et al., 2014).

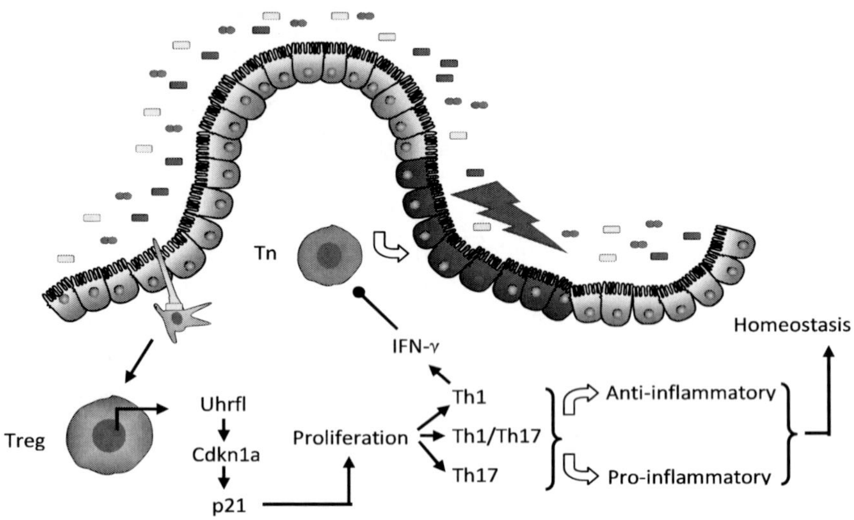

Figure 3. Influence of microbiota to Treg functioning. Sampling and presentation of microbiotal antigens by dendritic cells to regulatory T (Treg) cells activates transcription factors Uhrfl, Cdkn1a and p21. The later induces proliferation of effector T cells that increases production of anti-inflammatory cytokines and decreases that of pro-inflammatory cytokines leading to immune homeostasis. The signalling also increases production of interferon (IFN)-γ that downregulates production of naïve T cell to suppress inflammation in a disrupted microbiota environment.

Specific members of the intestinal microbiota have been shown to induce development of Foxp3$^+$ Treg cells. They do this via distinct mechanisms. *B. breve* induces development of IL-10-producing Tr1 cells that express cMaf, IL-21, and Ahr in the large intestine. This process is mediated by intestinal CD103$^+$ DCs which are activated by *B. breve* to produce IL-10 and IL-27 via toll-like receptor (TLR)/myeloid differentiation primary response gene (MyD)88 pathway (Figure 4). The produced IL-10-producing Tr1 cells can ameliorate colitis in immunocompromised mice (Jeon et al., 2012). A human commensal, *Bacteroides fragilis* and its products induce development of Foxp3$^+$ Treg cells in the large intestine. The commensal produces capsular polysaccharide-A moiety that mediates interaction of *B. fragilis* with the colonic mucosa to facilitate both colonization and activation of an anti-inflammatory response and promote expansion of colonic IL-10-expressing

Foxp3$^+$ Treg cells. The *B. fragilis* mediates these responses through TLR-2 MyD88 pathway (Round et al., 2011). Another modulation of Treg cells is by an altered Schaedler flora (ASF) that consists of eight species of the microbiota dominated by *Bacteroides distasonis*, but devoid of *B. fragilis*. This mixture induces expansion of Treg cells following colonization of germ-free mice (Geuking et al., 2011). Further studies have shown that the altered ASF leads to inappropriate expansion of colonic Th17 cells (Mosconi et al., 2013). These observations suggest that although certain components of the microbiota promote Treg-cell development, this phenomenon is not unique to any one microbial component and is not species specific. Indeed, this kind of redundant response is a suitable adaptive mechanism to ensure gut immunity. Additionally, intestinal colonization by *Clostridium* species triggers a TLR-independent, TGF-β-mediated induction of Foxp3$^+$ Treg cells in the large intestine. Expansion of Treg cells in the colons of germ-free mice can be achieved by a cocktail of *Clostridium* species comprised of clusters IV and XIVa. These species elicit production of TGF-β in the intestinal mucosa through enigmatic mechanisms (Atarashi et al., 2011).

In general terms, the microbiota-dependent induction of Foxp3$^+$ Treg cells is essential for the establishment of intestinal CD4$^+$ T cell homeostasis. Further, the microbiota educates Foxp3$^+$ Treg cells to acquire the antigen-specific repertoires of their T cell receptors (Lathrop et al., 2011). Through the antigen specific receptor repertoires, the microbiota influences gut homing of Treg cells. A recent study showed that colonic homing of Foxp3$^+$ Treg cells is mediated by guanine nucleotide-binding protein (G protein)-coupled receptor (GR)15 which is controlled by gut microbiota and TGF-β1. Mice deficient in GR15 fail to control infiltration of inflammatory cells to the colon lamina propria leading to severe colitis (Kim et al., 2013).

NKT CELLS

Gut NKT mediate their functions through production of various cytokines including GM-CSF, IFN-γ, IL-2, IL-4, IL-13, IL-17, IL-21, and TNF-α. Production of these cytokines is pivotal to instituting antimicrobial defense, cancer immunosurveillance and modulation of immune-mediated diseases by promoting or suppressing immune responses (Bouma and Strober 2003). NKT cells express NK1.1 molecules and can be grouped in type 1 (invariant) and type 2 NKT cells. Invariant NKT (iNKT) cells are classical NKT cells

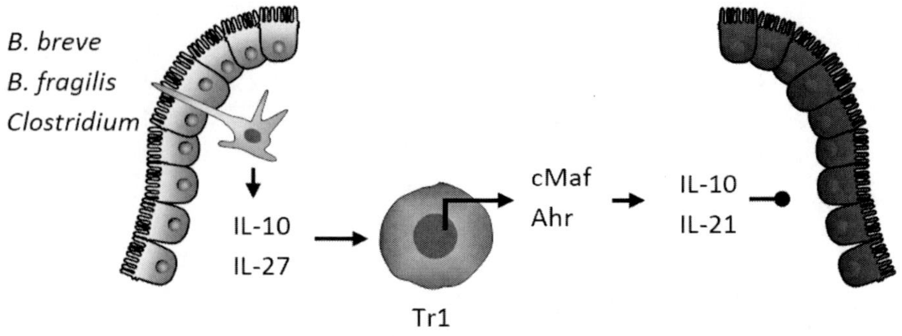

Figure 4. Influence of specific microbiota members to Treg during health and disease. Specific microbiota members like *Bifidobacterium breve, B. fragilis* and *Clostidium* spp induce production of mediators such as interleukin (IL)-10 and 27 that drives regulatory T (Tr1) cell to express cMaf and Ahr (aryl hydrocarbon receptor). This expression leads to production of IL-10 and IL-21 that curbs intestinal inflammation.

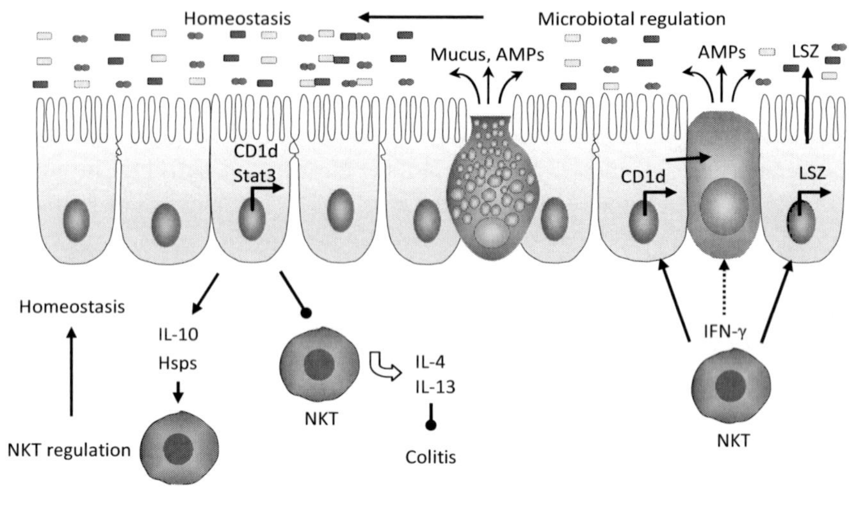

Figure 5. NKT cells and microbiota during homeostasis and disease. By activating intestinal CD1d, the microbiota activates Stat3 leading to production of anti-inflammatory mediators like heat shock proteins (Hsps) and interleukin (IL)-10. These mediators regulate NKT (natural killer T) cells leading to homeostasis. Stat3 activation also suppresses IL-4 and IL-13 production by NKT cells to ameliorate colitis. NKT cells can mimic interferon (IFN)-γ profile or activate CD1d to induce production of antimicrobial peptides (AMPs) by Paneth cells. They can also activate release of lysozymes (LSZ) by intestinal epithelial cells. The production of both AMPs and LSZ regulate the microbiota and maintains intestinal immunity.

expressing invariant T cell receptor α (TCR-α) chain. In addition, iNKT cells express and respond to transcriptional regulator promyelocytic leukemia zinc finger (PLZF) for development (Kovalovsky et al., 2008; Savage et al., 2008). The iNKT cells can differentiate into killer TFH cells and can support antibody response in germinal centers (Chang et al., 2012).

INFLUENCE OF MICROBIOTA TO NKT CELLS DURING HEALTH AND DISEASE

The interaction between microbiota and NKT cells has been reported by several researchers. It may involve cross-regulation between NKT cells and intestinal microbiota as well as epithelial CD1d molecule. The microbiota regulates intestinal NKT cell trafficking and function during postnatal life. Disruption of microbiota perturbs the microbiota-NKT cell interaction and predisposes to NKT cell-mediated diseases (Zeissig and Blumberg 2013).

Studies comparing NKT cells in animals harboring different microbiota profiles have shown that iNKT cell phenotype is affected by intestinal microbes. Different specified pathogen free (SPF) mice with different microbiota composition exhibit phenotypic variations in iNKT cell receptor Vβ7 frequency and cytokine profile. Those from germ-free mice show less maturity and decreased responsiveness to antigens. These attributes are corrected upon exposure to microbiota species containing iNKT cell antigens such as *Sphingomonas* (Wingender et al., 2012), indicating that the presence of glycolipids from the microbiota that is detected by epithelial CD1d and presented to iNKT cells drives the iNKT cell phenotype. This microbiota-driven phenotype has significant impact on gut homeostasis since germ-free animals experience high levels of iNKT cells in the colonic LP. The changes are associated with increased chemokine ligand CXCL16 and production of IL-4 and IL-13 that contribute to inflammatory reaction during ulcerative colitis (Bouma and Strober 2003). Such animals show high immune mobidity in various conditions including IBD (Olszak et al., 2012). Colonization with conventional microbiota ameliorates the mucosal increase in iNKT cells and treats the colitis (Olszak et al., 2012). Indeed, the microbiota shaping of iNKT cell phenotype is part and parcel of gut immunity.

Besides driving iNKT cell phenotype, the microbiota is also required for the development of iNKT cells. This is supported by the fact that germ-free animals have a moderately reduced number of these cells compared to conventional animals (Wei et al., 2010). Mice models of restricted flora (with preferential *Firmicutes* phylotype) have severe depletion of iNKT cells due to deficiency of *Sphingomonas* spp and their antigenic glycosphingolipid products. In addition, the restricted microbiota in these animals increases the number of $CD8^+$ Tc cells that suppress further the production of iNKT cells (Wei et al., 2010).

Recent studies have found that the NKT cell immunity follows activation from CD1d on the epithelial cells but not from bone marrow cells. The NKT protective responses are generated after engaging intestinal epithelial CD1d signaling. The signaling activates intestinal epithelial CD1d, Stat3, IL-10 and heat shock protein (Hsp) 110 production which play role in controlling intestinal inflammation. Depletion of any of these epithelial elements leads to severe NKT cell-mediated colitis (Olszak et al., 2014).

A cross-regulatory effect of NKT cells to the microbiota, mediated through Paneth cell products, has been observed. It is putatively known that Paneth cells can be activated by several means including cytokines like INF-γ to secrete bactericidal products from their granules (Malago 2014). The secreted products regulate the gut microbiota (Nieuwenhuis et al., 2009). It has recently been shown that iNKT cells recapitulate IFN-γ-dependent stimulation of Paneth cells to degranulate and release their chemicals. In so doing, the iNKT cells contribute to regulation of microbiota profile in the intestine (Farin et al., 2014). It is interesting to note that NKT cells induce release of lysozyme from intestinal crypts and that the NKT cell-specific epithelial CD1d molecules affect Paneth cell degranulation (Nieuwenhuis et al., 2009). Both events contribute significantly to the regulation of intestinal microbiota colonization and subsequent immunity (Figure 5).

Influence of Microbiota on Memory T Cells

Although literature is scarce on the effect of microbiota to memory T cells, there is enough evidence that the microbiota plays role in the expansion and function of memory T cells. This ability was demonstrated by Tanaka and colleagues who administered (intraperitoneal) murine cytomegalovirus to specific-pathogen free (SPF) or germ-free mice and observed a high cytomegalovirus-specific $CD8^+$ memory T cells in SPF animals. Reconstitution of microbiota in germ-free mice by oral administration of fecal suspension from SPF animals restores the $CD8^+$ memory T cells in these animals (Tanaka et al., 2007).

It has further been shown that activation and expansion of memory T cells is enhanced in the absence of microbiota. Mittrücker and colleagues observed that the lack of mirobiota in germ-free mice leads to high susceptibility and disease during *Listeria monocytogenes* infection. This infection triggers development of strong antilisterial CD8$^+$ memory T cells that clear bacteria during secondary infection more rapidly in germ-free than conventional animals (Mittrücker et al., 2014). It has also been shown that during primary infection, the gut immune tolerance to commensals is lost as microbiota-specific T cells differentiate to become inflammatory effector T cells as well as memory T cells. This parallel response spares the microbiota while destroying the pathogens (Hand et al., 2012).

The microbiota-memory T cell relationship on cancer cells has also been observed. It involves shaping anticancer immune responses by inducing memory Th1 cells. This occurs following administration of anticancer cyclophosphamide which disrupts intestinal microbiota. The disrupted microbiota leads to translocation of some Gram-positive bacteria into secondary lymphoid organs and induce generation of memory Th1 cells. Germ-free mice and those lacking Gram-positive commensal bacteria show low numbers of memory T cells and their tumors do not respond to cyclophosphamide (Viaud et al., 2013).

CONCLUSION

It is evident that the microbiota plays a pivotal role in shaping intestinal T cell functioning. This role is so critical that impairment of microbiota profile leads to diseases that can be cured on restoring the normal microbiotal profile. This is manifested by the role of effector T cells to drive gut inflammations through production of their pro-inflammatory cytokines. Maneuvers that suppress production of effector T cell cytokines can ameliorate severity of intestinal diseases. Such maneuvers may mimic effect of Treg cells that downregulate T effector cell functions. They may involve maintenance of normal microbiotal profile that influences optimal Treg functioning. The mechanisms involved in such therapy revolve around exploiting the anti-inflammatory role of microbiota-induced Treg cells to annul T effector functions. Although employment of Treg cells as therapeutics against intestinal disorders caused by disruption of intestinal microbiota such as IBD is not yet in place, there is a strong indication that they can curb such diseases. Apart from Treg cells, the expressed potential of iNKT and memory T cells in overcoming colitis (Olszak et al., 2014), infections (Mittrücker et al., 2014), and cancers (Viaud et al., 2013) is another indication that improvement of intestinal microbiota is essential for maintaining immunity. More research is needed to explore the therapeutic potential of microbiota-T cell interaction against intestinal disorders.

References

Arpaia, N; Campbell, C; Fan, X; et al. Metabolites produced by commensal bacteria promote peripheral regulatory T-cell *Nature.*, 2013, 504, 451-455.

Atarashi, K; Tanoue, T; Shima, T; et al. Induction of colonic regulatory T cells by indigenous Clostridium species. *Science.*, 2011, 331, 337-341.

Bouma, G; Strober, W. The immunological and genetic basis of inflammatory bowel disease. *Nat Rev Immunol*, 2003, 3, 521-533

Cao, AT; Yao, S; Gong, B; et al. Th17 cells upregulate polymeric Ig receptor and intestinal IgA and contribute to intestinal homeostasis. *J Immunol.*, 2012, 189, 4666-4673.

Carvalho, FA; Aitken, JD; Vijay-Kumar, M; et al. Toll-like receptor-gut microbiota interactions: perturb at your own risk! *Annu Rev Physiol.*, 2012, 74, 177-198.

Cebula, A; Seweryn, M; Rempala, GA; et al. Thymus-derived regulatory T cells contribute to tolerance to commensal microbiota. *Nature.*, 2013, 497, 258-262.

Chae, CS; Kwon, HK; Hwang, JS; et al. Prophylactic effect of probiotics on the development of experimental autoimmune myasthenia gravis. *PLoS One.*, 2012, 7, e52119.

Chang, PP; Barral, P; Fitch, J; et al. Identification of Bcl-6-dependent follicular helper NKT cells that provide cognate help for B cell responses. *Nat Immunol*, 2012, 13, 35–43.

Chappert, P; Bouladoux, N; Naik, S; et al. Specific gut commensal flora locally alters T cell tuning to endogenous ligands. *Immunity.*, 2013, 38, 1198-1210.

Chtanova, T; Tangye, SG; Newton, R; et al. T follicular helper cells express a distinctive transcriptional profile, reflecting their role as non-Th1/Th2 effector cells that provide help for B cells. *J Immunol.*, 2004, 173, 68-78.

Chung, Y; Tanaka, S; Chu, F; et al. Follicular regulatory T cells expressing Foxp3 and Bcl-6 suppress germinal center reactions. *Nat Med.*, 2011, 17, 983-988.

Curotto, de, Lafaille, MA; Lafaille, JJ. Natural and adaptive foxp3+ regulatory T cells: more of the same or a division of labor? *Immunity.*, 2009, 30, 626-635.

Evrard, B; Coudeyras, S; Dosgilbert, A; et al. Dose-dependent immunomodulation of human dendritic cells by the probiotic Lactobacillus rhamnosus Lcr35. *PLoS One.*, 2011, 6, e18735.

Farin, HF; Karthaus, WR; Kujala, P; et al. Paneth cell extrusion and release of antimicrobial products is directly controlled by immune cell-derived IFN-γ. *J Exp Med.*, 2014, 211, 1393-1405.

Fazilleau, N; Mark, L; McHeyzer-Williams, LJ; et al. Follicular helper T cells: lineage and location. *Immunity.*, 2009, 30, 324-335.

Feng, T; Cao, AT; Weaver, CT; et al. Interleukin-12 converts Foxp3+ regulatory T cells to interferon-γ-producing Foxp3+ T cells that inhibit colitis. *Gastroenterology.*, 2011, 140, 2031-2043

Feng, T; Elson, CO. Adaptive immunity in the host-microbiota dialog. *Mucosal Immunol.*, 2011, 4, 15-21.

Gaboriau-Routhiau, V; Rakotobe, S; Lécuyer, E; et al. The key role of segmented filamentous bacteria in the coordinated maturation of gut helper T cell responses. *Immunity.*, 2009, 31, 677-689.

Garrett, WS; Gallini, CA; Yatsunenko, T; et al. Enterobacteriaceae act in concert with the gut microbiota to induce spontaneous and maternally transmitted colitis. *Cell Host Microbe.*, 2010, 8, 292-300.

Geem, D; Medina-Contreras, O; McBride, M; et al. Specific microbiota-induced intestinal Th17 differentiation requires MHC class II but not GALT and mesenteric lymph nodes. *J Immunol.*, 2014, 193, 431-438.

Geuking, MB; Cahenzli, J; Lawson, MA; et al. Intestinal bacterial colonization induces mutualistic regulatory T cell responses. *Immunity.*, 2011, 34, 794-806.

Glatman, Zaretsky, A; Taylor, JJ; King, IL; et al. T follicular helper cells differentiate from Th2 cells in response to helminth antigens. *J Exp Med.*, 2009, 206, 991-999.

Hand, TW; Dos, Santos, LM; Bouladoux, N; et al. Acute gastrointestinal infection induces long-lived microbiota-specific T cell responses. *Science.*, 2012, 337, 1553-1556.

Hansen, CH; Andersen, LS; Krych, L; et al. Mode of delivery shapes gut colonization pattern and modulates regulatory immunity in mice. *J Immunol.*, 2014, 193, 1213-1222.

Hrncir, T; Stepankova, R; Kozakova, H; et al. Gut microbiota and lipopolysaccharide content of the diet influence development of regulatory T cells: studies in germ-free mice. *BMC Immunol.*, 2008, 9, 65

Ivanov, II; Atarashi, K; Manel, N; et al. Induction of intestinal Th17 cells by segmented filamentous bacteria. *Cell.*, 2009, 139, 485-498.

Ivanov, II; Frutos, Rde, L; Manel, N; et al. Specific microbiota direct the differentiation of IL-17-producing T-helper cells in the mucosa of the small intestine. *Cell Host Microbe.*, 2008, 4, 337-349.

Jakobsson, HE; Abrahamsson, TR; Jenmalm, MC; et al. Decreased gut microbiota diversity, delayed Bacteroidetes colonisation and reduced Th1 responses in infants delivered by caesarean section. *Gut.*, 2014, 63, 559-566.

Kim, CH. Host and microbial factors in regulation of T cells in the intestine. *Front Immunol.*, 2013, 4, 141.

Kim, SV; Xiang, WV; Kwak, C; et al. GPR15-mediated homing controls immune homeostasis in the large intestine mucosa. *Science.*, 2013, 340, 1456-1459.

Konieczna, P; Ferstl, R; Ziegler, M; et al. Immunomodulation by Bifidobacterium infantis 35624 in the murine lamina propria requires retinoic acid-dependent and independent mechanisms. *PLoS One.*, 2013, 8, e62617.

Kovalovsky, D; Uche, OU; Eladad, S; et al. The BTB-zinc finger transcriptional regulator PLZF controls the development of invariant natural killer T cell effector functions. *Nat Immunol.*, 2008, 9, 1055-1064.

Kwon, HK; Lee, CG; So, JS; et al. Generation of regulatory dendritic cells and CD4+Foxp3+ T cells by probiotics administration suppresses immune disorders. *Proc Natl Acad Sci U S A.*, 2010, 107, 2159-2164.

Lathrop, SK; Bloom, SM; Rao, SM; et al. Peripheral education of the immune system by colonic commensal microbiota. *Nature.*, 2011, 478, 250-254.

Linterman, MA; Pierson, W; Lee, SK; et al. Foxp3+ follicular regulatory T cells control the germinal center response. *Nat Med.*, 2011, 17, 975-982.

Maynard, CL; Elson, CO; Hatton, RD; et al. Reciprocal interactions of the intestinal microbiota and immune system. *Nature.*, 2012, 489, 231-241.

McGuckin, MA; Lindén, SK; Sutton, P; et al. Mucin dynamics and enteric pathogens. *Nat Rev Microbiol.*, 2011, 9, 265–278.

Mittrücker, HW; Seidel, D; Bland, PW; et al. Lack of microbiota reduces innate responses and enhances adaptive immunity against Listeria monocytogenes infection. *Eur J Immunol.*, 2014, 44, 1710-1715.

Mosconi, I; Geuking, MB; Zaiss, MM; et al. Intestinal bacteria induce TSLP to promote mutualistic T-cell responses. *Mucosal Immunol.*, 2013, 6, 1157-1167.

Mosmann, TR; Coffman, RL. TH1 and TH2 cells: different patterns of lymphokine secretion lead to different functional properties. *Annu Rev Immunol.*, 1989, 7, 145-173.

Nieuwenhuis, EE; Matsumoto, T; Lindenbergh, D; et al. Cd1d-dependent regulation of bacterial colonization in the intestine of mice. *J Clin Invest.*, 2009, 119, 1241-1250.

Nurieva, RI; Chung, Y; Hwang, D; et al. Generation of T follicular helper cells is mediated by interleukin-21 but independent of T helper 1, 2, or 17 cell lineages. *Immunity.*, 2008, 29, 138-149.

Obata, Y; Furusawa, Y; Endo, TA; et al. The epigenetic regulator Uhrf1 facilitates the proliferation and maturation of colonic regulatory T cells. *Nat Immunol.*, 2014, 15, 571-579.

Olszak, T; An, D; Zeissig, S; et al. Microbial exposure during early life has persistent effects on natural killer T cell function. *Science.*, 2012, 336, 489-493.

Olszak, T; Neves, JF; Dowds, CM; et al. Protective mucosal immunity mediated by epithelial CD1d and IL-10. *Nature.*, 2014, 509, 497-502.

Round, JL; Lee, SM; Li, J; et al. The Toll-like receptor 2 pathway establishes colonization by a commensal of the human microbiota. *Science.*, 2011, 332, 974-977.

Salzman, NH; Hung, K; Haribhai, D; et al. Enteric defensins are essential regulators of intestinal microbial ecology. *Nat Immunol.*, 2010, 11, 76-83.

Savage, AK; Constantinides, MG; Han, J; et al. The transcription factor PLZF directs the effector program of the NKT cell lineage. *Immunity.*, 2008, 29, 391-403.

Sawa, S; Lochner, M; Satoh-Takayama, N; et al. RORγt+ innate lymphoid cells regulate intestinal homeostasis by integrating negative signals from the symbiotic microbiota. *Nat Immunol.*, 2011, 12, 320-326.

Schiavi, E; Barletta, B; Butteroni, C; et al. Oral therapeutic administration of a probiotic mixture suppresses established Th2 responses and systemic anaphylaxis in a murine model of food allergy. *Allergy.*, 2011, 66, 499-508.

Sekirov, I; Russell, SL; Antunes, LC; et al. Gut microbiota in health and disease. *Physiol Rev.*, 2010, 90, 859-904.

Seo, GY; Youn, J; Kim, PH. IL-21 ensures TGF-beta 1-induced IgA isotype expression in mouse Peyer's patches. *J Leukoc Biol.*, 2009, 85, 744-750.

Shaw, MH; Kamada, N; Kim, YG; et al. Microbiota-induced IL-1β, but not IL-6, is critical for the development of steady-state TH17 cells in the intestine. *J Exp Med.*, 2012, 209, 251-258.

Tanaka, K; Sawamura, S; Satoh, T; et al. Role of the indigenous microbiota in maintaining the virus-specific CD8 memory T cells in the lung of mice infected with murine cytomegalovirus. *J Immunol.*, 2007, 178, 5209-5216.

Tap, J; Mondot, S; Levenez, F; et al. Towards the human intestinal microbiota phylogenetic core. *Environ Microbiol.*, 2009, 11, 2574-2584.

Viaud, S; Saccheri, F; Mignot, G; et al. The intestinal microbiota modulates the anticancer immune effects of cyclophosphamide. *Science.*, 2013, 342, 971-976.

Weaver, CT; Hatton, RD. Interplay between the TH17 and TReg cell lineages: a (co-)evolutionary perspective. *Nat Rev Immunol.*, 2009, 9, 883-889.

Wei, B; Wingender, G; Fujiwara, D; et al. Commensal microbiota and CD8+ T cells shape the formation of invariant NKT cells. *J Immunol.*, 2010, 184, 1218-1226.

Weiss, G; Rasmussen, S; Nielsen, Fink, L; et al. Bifidobacterium bifidum actively changes the gene expression profile induced by Lactobacillus acidophilus in murine dendritic cells. *PLoS One.*, 2010, 5, e11065.

Willinger, T; Freeman, T; Hasegawa, H; et al. Molecular signatures distinguish human central memory from effector memory CD8 T cell subsets. *J Immunol.*, 2005, 175, 5895-5903.

Wingender, G; Stepniak, D; Krebs, P; et al. Intestinal microbes affect phenotypes and functions of invariant natural killer T cells in mice. *Gastroenterology.*, 2012, 143, 418-428.

Yang, Y; Torchinsky, MB; Gobert, M; et al. Focused specificity of intestinal TH17 cells towards commensal bacterial antigens. *Nature.*, 2014, 510, 152-156.

Zeissig, S; Blumberg, RS. Commensal microbiota and NKT cells in the control of inflammatory diseases at mucosal surfaces. *Curr Opin Immunol.*, 2013, 25, 690-696.

ABOUT THE AUTHOR

Dr. Joshua Joseph Malago
Faculty of Veterinary Medicine
Sokoine University of Agriculture
P.O. Box 3203 Chuo Kikuu Morogoro Tanzania
Tel: +255 755 385610
malagojj@yahoo.com
malagojj@gmail.com
jmalago@suanet.ac.tz

INDEX

B

C

D

E

F

G

H

I

J

K

L

M

N

O

P

R

S

T